P

The
Peanut
Butter
Diet

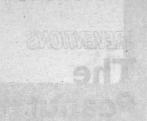

PREVENTION'S
The
Peanut
Butter
Diet

THE AMAZING EATING PLAN
THAT LETS YOU

- Lose Weight
- Lower Your Cholesterol
- Slash Your Risk of Heart
  Disease and Diabetes

HOLLY McCORD, M.A., R.D.
Nutrition Editor, *Prevention* Magazine

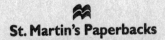

St. Martin's Paperbacks

THE PEANUT BUTTER DIET

Copyright © 2001 by Rodale Inc.

Prevention is a registered trademark of Rodale Inc.

ISBN: 0-312-98224-0

Printed in the United States of America

Recipe coordinator: Regina Ragone, R.D.
Menu development: Colleen Pierre, R.D., and Janis Jibrin, M.S., R.D.

Rodale/St. Martin's Paperbacks edition published August 2001

St. Martin's Paperbacks are published by St. Martin's Press, 175 Fifth Avenue, New York, NY 10010.

10 9 8 7 6 5 4 3 2 1

Visit us on the Web at www.prevention.com

NOTICE

This book is intended as a reference volume only, not as a medical manual. The information given here is designed to help you make informed decisions about your health and weight-loss needs. It is not intended as a substitute for any treatment or dietary advice that may have been prescribed by your doctor. If you suspect that you have a medical problem, we urge you to seek competent medical help. If you have not participated in an exercise program regularly or recently, we encourage you to work with your physician to determine the activity level that is best for you.

Mention of specific companies, organizations, or authorities in this book does not imply endorsement by the publisher, nor does mention of specific companies, organizations, or authorities in the book imply that they endorse the book.

Internet addresses and telephone numbers given in this book were accurate at the time this book went to press.

CONTENTS

ACKNOWLEDGMENTS

So many wonderful and talented people have helped transform the Peanut Butter Diet from a glimmer of an idea into the book you're holding in your hands. In particular, I want to recognize and thank Rodale president Steve Murphy, who realized before anyone that "The Amazing Peanut Butter Diet" (*Prevention*, March 2001) had even greater potential; senior vice president Marc Jaffe and subsidiary rights manager Dana Bacher, who found the book a home; lead researcher Karen Jacob, whose intrepid fact-finding skills made my job much easier; Colleen Pierre, R.D., and Janis Jibrin, M.S., R.D., who created the menu plans that are the foundation of the diet; *Prevention* food editor Regina Ragone, R.D., who helped coordinate the recipes; Rodale Test Kitchen manager JoAnn Brader, who helped make sure that every recipe is healthy and delicious; *Prevention* copy chief Linda Hager, who whipped the menu plans and recipes into shape; and *Prevention* fitness editor Michele Stanten, who graciously shared her knowledge of exercise and weight loss.

Thank you, too, to Rodale Women's Health Books editor-in-chief Tammerly Booth, whose vision helped shape the contents of the book; editor Susan Berg, who managed the manuscript with the patience of an angel; research managers Anita Small and Shea Zukowski, who performed a small miracle in pushing the entire manuscript through fact checking in a week; researchers Molly

Brown, Christine Dreisbach, Jennifer Goldsmith, Elizabeth Price, Sally Reith, Lisa Vroman, and Teresa Yeykal, whose tremendous grace under pressure made fact checking review a breeze; managing editor Madeleine Adams, who guided the manuscript through a demanding schedule; and senior copyeditor Jane Sherman, whose attention to detail polished the text.

The entire staff of *Prevention* magazine helped see me through this project, whether by offering words of encouragement or taking on an extra assignment so I could keep on writing. Special thanks go to editor-in-chief Catherine Cassidy, senior features editor Denise Foley, and assistant nutrition editor Gloria McVeigh, who allowed me to set aside my editorial duties for 2 full months; and research director Susan Coenen, who made sure I had the research support I needed from day one.

Finally, I want to thank Heather Jackson, editor at St. Martin's Press, for her perceptive suggestions in fine-tuning the manuscript, and Pat Kearney, director of The Peanut Institute, for her invaluable assistance in navigating the monounsaturated minefield. Without them, and without every person mentioned above, this book simply would not exist.

INTRODUCTION

Eat rich, delicious peanut butter and lose weight?

I admit, the Peanut Butter Diet sounds a little gim-
micky. Like the Cabbage Soup Diet, only worse—because it entices you to slim down by indulging in one of
the most calorie-dense foods around.

Make no mistake: If you decide to try the Peanut Butter Diet, you're embarking on a very controversial eating
plan.

Unlike the low-fat, high-carbohydrate diets that have
been endorsed by nutrition experts for years—and that
continue to be a very healthy choice for many people—
the Peanut Butter Diet delivers a higher proportion (about
35 percent) of its calories as fat. Most of that fat is the
healthy monounsaturated kind found in peanut butter.

Diets higher in monounsaturated fat have already won
support within the mainstream medical community as being very good for heart health. For proof, you need look
no further than the updated dietary guidelines released in
May 2001 by the National Cholesterol Education Program of the National Institutes of Health. For the first
time, these guidelines describe a heart-friendly diet as
one that gets up to 35 percent of its calories from fat—
provided that it's mostly unsaturated fat, including the
monounsaturated kind.

As far as your heart goes, what's most important is
keeping your intake of saturated fat—from foods like

meat, butter, and cheese—as low as possible. And of course, *not* gaining weight.

That's where the Peanut Butter Diet becomes controversial. Peanut butter packs a whopping 190 calories in every 2-tablespoon serving, so working more peanut butter, or more of any healthy fat, into your diet without putting on pounds can be tricky. And that is certainly cause for concern. After all, more than half of Americans are now overweight, a national health crisis to be sure. Weighing more than you should is bad for your heart and for most of the rest of your body, too.

So, won't you inevitably get heavier if you eat more fat, even a good fat like peanut butter? Right now, a lot of weight-loss experts are totally convinced that's exactly what will happen. "If you tell Americans to eat more fat, they'll wind up getting even fatter than they already are!" they say. I used to say that, too.

But my new hunch is that you *won't* gain weight—and a growing number of my colleagues would agree. We're basing our argument on a groundbreaking 18-month study presented at the 1999 Experimental Biology conference in Washington, D.C. For the study, researchers assigned two groups of people—all overweight—to follow two different diets. One was the standard low-fat, high-carbohydrate eating plan that's usually recommended for weight loss; the other was a high-monounsaturated-fat, moderate-carbohydrate eating plan that included peanut butter. Everyone in the study met with dietitians for counseling about calorie control.

By the end of this fascinating study, more than three times as many people in the high-monounsaturated-fat group had taken pounds off and kept them off, the hardest part of any weight-control program. In other words, eating more fat—some in the form of rich, satisfying peanut butter—made people thinner rather than heavier. That's revolutionary! The authors of the study believe, and I agree, that the people who ate a high-monounsaturated-fat diet were able to maintain calorie control because their diet tasted better. I suspect future studies will support this important finding.

In the meantime, so that you may experience the same weight-loss benefits that the folks in the study enjoyed, I've created the Peanut Butter Diet. It's designed to take off ½ pound a week by allowing for satisfying portions of peanut butter but still controlling calories.

You'll get 4 tablespoons of peanut butter a day if you're a woman, 6 tablespoons a day if you're a man. You'll enjoy treats like peanut butter whipped into a shake, peanut butter stirred into oatmeal, and peanut butter spread on a toasted English muffin. They're incorporated into menu plans that also provide for nine servings of fruits and vegetables a day. The menus are incredibly healthy—and incredibly easy, designed to get you out of the kitchen fast.

Of course, the *real* secret to the Peanut Butter Diet—beyond its utter satisfaction and simplicity—is its portion control. Peanut butter is so high in calories that eating even a little more each day than the diet calls for can pack on pounds *fast*. That's exactly what many weight-loss experts predict will happen.

But if you need to slim down and you happen to love peanut butter, some preliminary research suggests that an eating plan like the Peanut Butter Diet may actually make weight loss and weight maintenance easier. (Wouldn't that confound the experts!) But please note: If you try this diet and you find yourself bingeing on peanut butter, *stop*. You may be better off giving peanut butter a wide berth, at least for now.

And don't forget that if weight loss is your goal, you absolutely must get your vitamin X, as in "x-ercise." According to the latest government guidelines, accumulating 45 minutes of physical activity every day is ideal. This doesn't mean that you need to head out for a run every morning. Just taking the stairs at every opportunity can help!

Everything that makes the Peanut Butter Diet work—from measuring peanut butter portions to preparing meals and snacks to getting enough physical activity—is spelled out in the chapters that follow. From one peanut butter lover to another, I wish you fabulous health and the weight loss you dream of!

PART I

Yes, You *Can* Lose Weight Eating Peanut Butter

CHAPTER ONE

It Only *Sounds* Too Good to Be True!

Ask anyone to name a food that can help melt away extra pounds, and it almost certainly wouldn't be peanut butter. Yogurt? Probably. Celery? Absolutely. But *peanut butter*?

I must admit, the very idea of slimming down while indulging in peanut butter seems unbelievable. Except for one thing: It can be done. I've got new research to prove it!

In the pages that follow, you'll find a delicious, fuss-free plan that shows how you can not only achieve the weight loss you want but also improve your health in ways you would never have expected. And you'll do it by enjoying America's favorite comfort food—twice a day!

NO LONGER OFF-LIMITS?

If you're like me, peanut butter is among the foods you crave the most. It's rich, it's sticky, it tastes like roasted peanuts. It's ready whenever you are. I'm such a fan that I carried a peanut butter and jelly sandwich to school almost every day from first grade through senior year (and woe to my poor mother if she ever ran out of the stuff!).

But then I grew up, and I had to face two eye-opening facts about peanut butter:

- All those calories! Peanut butter is, shall we say, very well endowed. Two tablespoons contains

190 calories (compared with, for instance, 2 tablespoons of applesauce, which has 22 calories). Eat too much peanut butter, and you will gain weight—very quickly.

- All that fat! A 2-tablespoon serving delivers 16 grams of fat—as much as in a whole hamburger from Burger King, for heaven's sake. In the 1970s and 1980s, scientists pinned the blame for heart disease on a too-high fat intake. We came to view any high-fat food as "bad," though we now know that to be an oversimplification.

AMERICA'S FAVORITE COMFORT FOOD

Every 5 years, Kraft Foods analyzes more than 1,700 households nationwide to find out what Americans are stocking in their kitchens. In 2000, out of 100 common food items, peanut butter came in fourth, with jars in 83 percent of kitchens. Only eggs, granulated sugar, and flour ranked higher. This may explain how we Americans manage to consume more than 700 million pounds of peanut butter annually!

In case you're curious, here's a rundown of the top 25 kitchen staples, as identified by the Kraft Foods survey:

1. Eggs	14. Barbecue sauce
2. Granulated sugar	15. Yellow onions
3. Flour	16. Spaghetti sauce
4. Peanut butter	17. Canned tomato sauce
5. Ground black pepper	18. Margarine
6. Ketchup	19. Idaho baking potatoes
7. Baking soda	(fresh)
8. Yellow mustard	20. Oregano
9. Vanilla extract	21. Corn
10. Baking powder	22. Hamburger
11. Ground cinnamon	23. Vegetable oil
12. Spaghetti/vermicelli	24. Saltines
13. Brown sugar	25. Bottled salad dressing

Regretfully, I felt I had no choice but to do what many peanut butter lovers have done: I put peanut butter on my taboo list. Except, of course, for the times I broke down and ate it right out of the jar with a spoon—a stealthy pleasure marred by tons of guilt. (I've since learned that this habit is a bad one, for a reason besides calorie overload. To learn more, see "The Surprising Danger of Spooning" below.)

THE SURPRISING DANGER OF SPOONING

If you eat peanut butter right out of the jar with a spoon, or even from your finger, you may want to change your ways. According to Henry Heimlich, M.D., creator of the Heimlich Maneuver and president of the Heimlich Institute at Deaconess Hospital in Cincinnati, "If a glob of peanut butter is eaten off a spoon, the peanut butter can be sucked into the airways and block them. In such instances, it spreads through the lungs." Dr. Heimlich recommends spreading peanut butter on bread or crackers before eating it.

Still, choking on peanut butter is not all that common, according to Richard O'Brien, M.D., emergency physician at Moses Taylor Hospital in Scranton, Pennsylvania, and spokesperson for the American College of Emergency Physicians. "Choking on a piece of meat that is too big or not chewed properly accounts for 99 percent of the cases we see in the ER," he says. "But if someone were choking on peanut butter, the first thing I'd do is the Heimlich Maneuver."

So if you're a "spooner," consider yourself warned! The good news is, with the meals and snacks in the Peanut Butter Diet, you'll discover lots of safe and delicious ways to indulge in peanut butter.

THANK YOU, SCIENCE!

Then some fabulous news about peanut butter started trickling in from nutrition research laboratories. True, peanut butter is high in fat. But most of it is monounsaturated, the same "good fat" that's found in olive oil. Groundbreaking studies were proving that a diet high in monounsaturated fat from peanuts and peanut butter could actually be good for the heart, and perhaps even better than the low-fat, high-carbohydrate diet most health experts were recommending. A diet high in monounsaturated fat even looked promising as a treatment for diabetes, a disease that has become epidemic in the United States.

But the best news was yet to come, especially for all those health-conscious peanut butter lovers whose biggest question was "If I eat more peanut butter, won't I pack on pounds?" The amazing answer turned out to be "Not necessarily!"

In fact, research conducted over the past few years suggests that going back to peanut butter may actually take off unwanted pounds more easily than following a standard low-fat eating plan. In one revealing experiment, almost three times as many peanut butter dieters as low-fat dieters managed to maintain their weight loss over an 18-month period. (You'll find out more about that research in chapter 2.)

> **DID YOU KNOW . . .**
>
> Six of the top 10 candy bars contain peanuts or peanut butter.
>
> SOURCE: THE NATIONAL PEANUT BOARD

But here's the hitch: Unless you're experienced in nutrition, designing an eating plan that packs in peanut butter plus all the nutrients you need without going overboard on calories can be extremely tricky. If you don't watch your calories, you will gain weight. A calorie is still a calorie. Eat more than you burn up, and watch that scale climb—fast.

So to help my fellow peanut butter lovers succeed in losing weight (and reap other health benefits besides), I—

with my colleagues at *Prevention* magazine—have created the Peanut Butter Diet. It's a super-delicious, supereasy 28-day plan that tells you exactly what to eat at every meal and snack so you can satisfy your craving for peanut butter while controlling calories. As a bonus, you'll help your heart and stock up on scarce nutrients.

Prevention published 5 days of the plan in its March 2001 issue, and readers begged for more. That's how this book was born.

SECRETS OF SUCCESS

Actually, the Peanut Butter Diet is two eating plans with different calorie intakes, one for women and the other for men. The diet works because it's based on two solid nutritional principles.

Portion control. We've carefully designed 4 weeks of ultra-satisfying menus to allow women two 2-tablespoon servings of peanut butter and men three 2-tablespoon servings, every day. (Because of their larger body size, men can eat a little more.) That's a nice, satisfying lump of peanut butter, but it's nestled into meals and snacks in ways that still control calories.

For the Peanut Butter Diet to be successful, though, you've got to stick with that 2-tablespoon serving. In chapter 8, I'll show you how you to quickly and easily measure out 2 tablespoons of peanut butter without resorting to measuring spoons. (Hint: It involves a Ping-Pong ball.)

Amazing satisfaction. Because the Peanut Butter Diet has more fat than the standard low-fat diet (but is at least as healthy, if not more so), and because it features America's favorite comfort food, you won't feel deprived. This means you have a better chance of staying with the plan and losing the weight you want.

According to Baltimore-based dietitian Colleen Pierre, R.D., dietary fat promotes satiety, the feeling of satisfaction after a meal. "I see many clients who've been following low-fat diets full of rice cakes and water, and they wonder why they're hungry all the time," she says. "I tell them to start including fat in their meals and snacks, and they stop feeling so starved."

Actually, peanut butter may be extra-satisfying. In his own research, Richard Mattes, R.D., Ph.D., associate professor of foods and nutrition at Purdue University in West Lafayette, Indiana, discovered that people who snacked on peanut butter self-adjusted their calorie intakes for the rest of the day. In other words, without being told what to do, they naturally ate fewer calories later on to come out roughly even for the day. They felt satisfied longer, too.

When participants in Dr. Mattes's study were fed a typical portion of other snacks, such as rice cakes, their hunger returned within a half-hour. After a snack of peanut butter, their hunger subsided for about 2½ hours.

EASY DOES IT BETTER

Here's another reason that you have a better chance of remaining faithful to the Peanut Butter Diet: The calorie intake has been calculated so that the average woman or man will take off about ½ pound per week, or a total of 25 pounds in a year.

Why not lose weight faster—say, 1 to 2 pounds a week, as some other diets promise? Because losing weight faster means cutting calories much lower. Sure, that works for a while, during what dietitians call the honeymoon period. But eventually, many people feel so deprived that they go back to overeating. The more gradually you slim down, the less deprived you'll feel. That's why the Peanut Butter Diet is your best bet for getting to your goal—and staying there.

HOW DEEP IS YOUR LOVE?

On prevention.com, the *Prevention* magazine Web site, we posed the following question: "Have you ever eaten peanut butter directly from the jar?" Here's how people responded.

2,735 said, "Yes, I spoon it directly into my mouth."

1,094 said, "Yes, I stick my finger right in the jar."

438 said, "No, I measure out careful servings."

403 said, "No, I hate peanut butter."

Are you worried that once you start eating peanut butter, you won't be able to stop? Dietitian Pierre says her clients often binge on peanut butter because they turn to it when they're half-starved. "One of my clients would skip breakfast, have a salad and diet soda for lunch, then eat half a jar of peanut butter after work," she says. "No wonder she couldn't stop. The poor thing was starving!"

But once her clients adopt a pattern of regular meals and snacks that include peanut butter, their urge to binge goes away, Pierre adds. Indeed, in a study reported at an Experimental Biology conference, Dr. Mattes and his colleagues found that getting people to add 500 calories' worth of peanuts to their daily diets over a 3-week period was difficult. "They commented that they were just too full!" he says.

That said, peanut butter can be a trigger food for some people. In other words, once they eat a little, they can hardly resist finishing off the jar. If this sounds like you, you'll want to read chapter 2, where I discuss this phenomenon in further detail.

WHEN ENOUGH IS ENOUGH

While some people—me, for instance—can indulge in peanut butter every day and not get tired of it, you may find that after eating two or three servings a day for several weeks, you're ready for a change. That's no problem. Simply switch to another balanced 1,500- or 2,200-calorie eating plan for a while. (The lower calorie cap is for women, the higher one for men.) I'll show you how to create your own menus, sans peanut butter, in chapter 14.

> **DID YOU KNOW . . .**
>
> Peanut butter was the secret behind Mister Ed, TV's talking horse. It made him move his mouth at the right times.
>
> SOURCE: THE NATIONAL PEANUT BOARD

Eventually, you may decide to return to the Peanut Butter Diet for another 4 weeks. Or you may just want to keep a few favorite menu plans handy so you won't blow your calorie budget the next time you need a peanut butter fix. But if you love peanut butter the way I do, I'm betting that you'll be back for good!

CHAPTER TWO

The Science behind the Diet

Overweight and obesity are the new American epidemic. Currently, less than half of us—about 45 percent—weigh what we should. *More* than half of us need to lose a few or quite a few pounds to avoid serious health risks.

In fact, one-quarter of Americans are more than 30 percent above their ideal weights, the point at which poor health consequences become a virtual certainty. But probably the first wish in most dieters' hearts is to slim down so they will look better. There's nothing wrong with that, either. It's a wonderful motivator.

Yet when I mention the Peanut Butter Diet to people, the first thing they say is, "It's impossible to eat peanut butter and lose weight!" Why? Because they know how high in calories peanut butter is. As I mentioned in chapter 1, 190 calories lurk in every 2-tablespoon serving. That's why the weight-conscious and the health-conscious tend to avoid peanut butter like the plague. But I suspect that some of them occasionally binge on it, too.

THE RESEARCH THAT STARTED IT ALL

Given peanut butter's reputation as a fattening food, why would anyone deliberately make it an ingredient in a weight-loss plan? Yet that's exactly what Kathy McManus, M.S., R.D., director of nutrition at Brigham and

WAY BEYOND LOOKING GOOD

Most of us who want to drop some extra pounds are driven by a desire to look better. If we succeed, our bodies will be a heck of a lot healthier, too.

In the United States, an estimated 97 million adults are considered overweight or obese (with obesity often defined as being more than 30 percent above a healthy weight). A National Institutes of Health (NIH) report says that "as a major cause of preventable death in the United States today, overweight and obesity pose a major public health challenge." In fact, they're second only to smoking as the nation's leading cause of preventable death.

According to the NIH, carrying extra pounds can substantially increase a person's risk of the following diseases.

- High blood pressure
- Heart disease
- Type 2 (non-insulin-dependent) diabetes
- Stroke
- Gallbladder disease
- Osteoarthritis
- Sleep apnea and other breathing problems
- Cancers of the uterine lining (endometrium), breast, prostate, and colon

In addition, people who are overweight may experience social stigmatization and discrimination—certainly unjustly so. But it is one of the reasons that carrying extra pounds raises the risk of depression.

The good news is, studies have shown that dropping even 5 to 10 pounds can have significant health benefits in terms of reducing high blood pressure, high blood sugar, and high cholesterol. So your best bet may be to lose a small amount of weight, in the 5- to 10-pound range, and to maintain that loss for a while. Once you've accomplished that, aim to shed another 5 to 10 pounds. Continue in increments until you reach your goal weight.

Women's Hospital in Boston, and Frank Sacks, M.D., professor of nutrition at Harvard School of Public Health, decided to do.

"It really grew out of our experiences with our patients," McManus explains. "We were seeing people one-on-one, and we found that some overweight individuals were unsuccessful at keeping pounds off for any length of time when they followed low-fat diets. We also noticed that when some patients went on low-fat diets, their triglycerides actually rose, and their good HDL cholesterol sometimes fell. Both changes can increase heart attack risk. This was back in 1993, just about the time the Mediterranean diet—rich in monounsaturated fat from olive oil—was getting a lot of attention in the United States."

A few years later, McManus and Dr. Sacks designed preliminary research to compare the effects of calorie-controlled moderate-fat and low-fat diets in obese adults. The surprising findings of their initial work were first presented at the 1999 Experimental Biology conference held in Washington, D.C. Their research suggests that calorie-controlled diets containing moderate amounts of fat, including peanut butter, could play a role in weight loss.

McManus and Dr. Sacks assigned 101 men and women—average weight 200 pounds—to one of two groups. Those in one group were instructed to limit their fat intake to a low 20 percent of calories. Those in the other group had a more generous fat allowance: 35 percent of calories, which came from foods rich in monounsaturated fat, such as peanut butter, nuts, olive oil, and avocados. Both groups kept a rein on foods high in saturated fat, such as red meat, cheese, and butter.

Once a week, the two groups met with registered dietitians, who counseled them in making food choices that would supply approximately 1,200 calories a day for the women and 1,500 calories a day for the men. But the study participants were what scientists call free-living. In other words, what they ate was really up to them. They also added regular exercise to their daily routines.

Many dietitians have noticed that getting people to buy into a moderate-fat diet like the one McManus and Dr. Sacks used is a lot more difficult than expected. "Even though my clients are overweight, they are used to steaming vegetables, sautéing with a little cooking spray, or using fat-free salad dressing," explains Jane Malyn, R.D., a nutrition therapist in suburban Philadelphia. "Convincing them to change their low-fat habits can be tough at first."

> **DID YOU KNOW . . .**
>
> Enough peanuts are grown on 1 acre to make 30,000 peanut butter sandwiches.
>
> SOURCE: THE NATIONAL
> PEANUT BOARD

But after a while, Malyn adds, her clients are very pleased that they can reintroduce foods rich in unsaturated fat into their diets. "Fat tastes good, no matter what," she says. "When you add a little bit to your vegetables or salads, you enjoy them more."

Of course, the big question is, did anyone involved in the preliminary research that McManus and Dr. Sacks conducted end up losing weight? In fact, everyone who remained in the program shed about the same number of pounds—11—during the first 3 to 6 months. As dietitians know, that's the "honeymoon period" during which most people can stick with any eating plan.

What's most revealing is that over the 18 months of the study, almost three times as many people stayed on the moderate-fat diet as on the low-fat diet. What's more, during the last 12 to 18 months, those who remained in the low-fat group gained back about 5 pounds, while those in the moderate-fat group kept off the total amount they had lost—11 pounds.

What made the difference? As McManus remarked in

Prevention's March 2001 issue, "Taste is first. People have to enjoy what they eat to stick with it." Although the research was not designed to look specifically at attitudes toward peanut butter, Malyn has noticed that when she gives clients a choice between incorporating more olive oil or more peanut butter into their diets, they choose peanut butter fairly quickly. That's because it's such a delightful substitution for what they have been eating.

"Instead of spreading fat-free margarine on their toast, they use peanut butter, which is a big treat," Malyn says. "And they loved being able to make a peanut butter sandwich. That's a very portable, very enjoyable lunch that many people miss."

My conclusion from the preliminary research and from dietitians' own experiences: For some people who want to slim down, a calorie-controlled, moderate-fat diet built around foods rich in monounsaturated fat—including peanut butter—may be easier to maintain. And that means your weight loss is more likely to be permanent.

MORE PROOF IN PEANUT BUTTER

Other researchers have tested a low-fat diet against a diet that got most of its fat from peanut butter and peanuts. They found that peanut butter is no barrier to losing weight.

At Pennsylvania State University in University Park, Penny Kris-Etherton, R.D., Ph.D., and Christine Pelkman, Ph.D., compared two small groups of overweight people, average age 44. For 6 weeks, one group followed a diet that provided 20 percent of its calories as fat, while the other group was assigned a diet that delivered 35 percent of its calories as fat—half of which came from peanuts and peanut butter. All the food for the study was prepared at the university. The calorie intake was tailored for each person so that it would produce about the same rate of weight loss in everyone.

After 6 weeks, both groups had shed an average of 15 pounds. But according to Dr. Kris-Etherton, "The people on the peanut diet said it was just so much better and so much easier to follow, without question. And they certainly ended up with better triglyceride profiles, despite losing the same amount of weight." (The study was reported at the April 2001 Experimental Biology meeting, held in San Diego.)

SO WHAT ABOUT LOW-FAT DIETS?

To be fair, some data indicate that people who follow low-fat diets are the most successful at keeping off weight. The National Weight Control Registry, affiliated with Colorado Health Sciences University in Denver, records the names of dieters who have lost 30 pounds or more and who have maintained that loss for at least a year. According to James Hill, Ph.D., one of the registry's directors, while people can slim down on many types of diets, 95 percent of those who shed pounds permanently do so by following low-fat, high-carbohydrate diets.

That's not hard to understand, Dr. Kris-Etherton says, since fat has 9 calories per gram, while carbohydrates have just 4 calories per gram. "I think the way this is netting out is to not go too high in total fat, because it can supply too many calories," she says. "But to go too *low* in total fat—that's restrictive and hard for some people to maintain. It can also raise triglycerides and blood sugar."

Every expert I spoke with identified one point as key to the success of the Peanut Butter Diet: careful portion control. "Distinct menu plans are a must," Dr. Pelkman says. "That way, people know exactly how many calories they are getting."

Malyn wholeheartedly agrees, emphasizing that "you can't just take a jar of peanut butter and go to town. If you're going to try a moderate-fat diet, you need to control calories. You can't get away from that."

As McManus and Dr. Sacks concluded, the value of their moderate-fat diet is that it's a tasty alternative to the usual weight-loss plans. Baltimore-based dietitian Colleen Pierre, R.D., agrees. "It's something that can be followed over the long term, as opposed to a diet that doesn't taste so good and that makes people want to get off it so they can go back to the foods they really want," she says. "That's what a lot of us do."

Pierre has been recommending a diet higher in monounsaturated fat to some of her clients, with impressive results. "I have one client who switched to this type of diet to lower his triglycerides," Pierre says. "He wasn't very heavy to begin with, but he lost a few pounds along the way. Months later, I ran into his wife, who just raved about his continued success in both keeping off the weight and lowering his triglycerides.

"I'm currently counseling a couple who started a diet high in monounsaturated fat to slim down and to control an array of health problems, including diabetes, high blood pressure, and sleep apnea," Pierre adds. "When they went on vacation, they actually lost weight. They're doing great!"

Pierre has put peanut butter to the test in her own life as well. Following the birth of her daughter, she shed some of her "baby fat" in part by having a peanut butter sandwich with carrot sticks and fat-free milk for lunch every day. "Every ongoing diet is a bit of a struggle," she says. "Including favorite foods is key to keeping your tastebuds happy, so you don't feel deprived."

As for Malyn, she has created her own peanut butter snack to satisfy her late-afternoon munchies. Her youngest daughter, Julie, takes peanut butter on whole wheat sandwiches to school. But she doesn't like the crusts, so she carries them home every day. Mom spreads them with peanut butter and finishes them off. "It's amazing how that little bit satisfies me," she says.

INDULGING WITHOUT OVERDOING

The Peanut Butter Diet offers moderate monounsaturated fat, adequate protein, slightly reduced carbohydrate, and tons of fiber, plus vitamins and minerals. If you follow the menu plans, you'll be getting just the right number of calories. So you can't overdo—theoretically.

But for some of us, peanut butter can be a trigger food. In other words, if we eat a little, we want even more. "The serving size for peanut butter is not the entire jar!" admonishes Leslie Bonci, M.P.H., R.D., director of nutrition at the University of Pittsburgh Center for Sports Medicine and spokesperson for the American Dietetic Association.

For those in danger of overdoing it, dietitian Pierre offers this sound advice: "If you're scared of peanut butter, you need to change your self-talk. Instead of thinking that peanut butter has always been your downfall and that as soon as you open the jar, you'll eat the whole thing, start telling yourself that you can eat peanut butter every day for the rest of your life—and still lose weight! Write it down if you need to, and post it on the refrigerator door. Tape a note on the peanut butter jar, too."

But what if you do slip and eat too much? "Try harder to break the cycle of bingeing and starving, but not by swearing off peanut butter forever. That's probably what got you in this jam in the first place," Pierre says. "Go back to your 4 or 6 tablespoons a day. Eventually, peanut butter will seem normal instead of naughty."

Should anyone avoid peanut butter for fear of binge-ing? "If opening that jar really terrifies you, maybe you should wait until you feel more confident about slimming down," says Pierre, who has counseled thousands of clients about weight loss. "It's a tough job to shed un-wanted pounds and keep them off. Having a positive mindset is key."

I couldn't agree more. If in 2 weeks on the Peanut But-ter Diet you find yourself going on peanut butter binges, *stop*! The last thing I want you to do is put on extra pounds, and I know it's the last thing you want, too. But don't be discouraged from trying other ways to slim down. Thomas Edison is credited with a wonderful quote that applies here: "I have not failed. I have just found 10,000 ways that won't work."

Just don't give up. Most of the people in the National Weight Control Registry who were successful at weight loss tried dieting several times before finally getting the hang of staying slim. My hunch is, if you hang in there, peanut butter can become a healthy, pleasurable part of your life.

NEVER TOO MUCH OF A GOOD THING

One of the mantras among nutrition experts is that variety is essential to a healthy diet. As a registered dietitian, I wholeheartedly agree. Different foods come packaged with different nutrients. Always building your meals around the same small group of foods is going to cheat you of vitamins, minerals, and other compounds you need.

So how can I recommend a diet in which so much of the monounsaturated fat comes from peanut butter? There are three reasons.

This is the American version of the Mediterranean diet, with peanut butter replacing olive oil. In the heart-healthy Mediterranean diet, most of the monounsaturated fat comes from olive oil. "But if Americans were advised to adopt Mediterranean-style eating habits, most wouldn't be clear on how to appropriately incorporate more olive oil into their meals. And some just don't like it," Dr. Kris-Etherton notes.

> **DID YOU KNOW . . .**
>
> Peanut butter was introduced in the United States in 1904 by C. H. Sumner, who sold $705.11 worth of the "new treat" at his concession stand at the World's Fair in St. Louis.
>
> SOURCE: THE NATIONAL PEANUT BOARD

So, instead of using olive oil as the source of monounsaturated fat, I'm recommending another source that most Americans love and can easily use: peanut butter.

This is a varied diet. If you follow the Peanut Butter Diet, you'll be getting at least nine servings a day of fruits and vegetables, plus whole grains, beans, fish and lean meat, and high-calcium foods. I'd be willing to bet it's got tons more variety than any diet you may be following right now.

You can easily switch to other monounsaturated fats. In all probability, even peanut butter fanatics will want a change after several weeks of eating peanut butter every day. That's to be expected. And that's why I'm giving you the formula to design your own meal plans using other sources of monounsaturated fat, like olive oil, olives, avocados, and other nuts, plus some menu ideas. (It's all explained in chapter 14. How about some guacamole on baked tortilla chips? Yum!) But in the meantime, you'll be adjusting to a pattern of eating that controls calories while incorporating higher levels of a healthy fat.

And when the urge to eat peanut butter strikes again? You'll be prepared with menu plans that help satisfy your peanut butter cravings without blowing your calorie budget. Go back to them for a day or two, a month or two, or as long as you like.

CHAPTER THREE

Who Should Follow the Peanut Butter Diet?

If you're a fan of peanut butter, you don't need a good reason to try the Peanut Butter Diet. Just getting to enjoy one of your favorite foods every day is enticing enough!

That said, some people may find the Peanut Butter Diet especially beneficial. We've already seen how it can support weight loss when traditional low-fat diets don't seem to work. Even if you're not overweight, you may relish the idea of indulging in peanut butter without putting on unwanted pounds. For you, the Peanut Butter Diet could be fun.

In addition, this diet may be able to help lower high triglycerides, manage diabetes, and control a cluster of symptoms known as Syndrome X. We'll talk more about each of these conditions in the following chapters.

Nevertheless, the Peanut Butter Diet isn't for everyone. Certain people may want or need to avoid peanut butter. So please be sure to read this chapter. Don't ever take chances with your body and your health that you don't have to.

THE RED FLAGS

As popular as peanut butter is, some people just shouldn't eat it. Steer clear if any of the following apply to you.

You're allergic to peanuts. Up to 1 percent of the U.S. population has peanut allergies. They're an obvious reason to avoid peanut butter or any other food containing peanut products. Peanuts are the leading cause of severe allergic reaction, or anaphylaxis. One of the key symptoms of anaphylaxis is a severe drop in blood pressure, which can prove fatal.

If you'd like to try a diet higher in monounsaturated fats, use olive oil and olives, avocados, canola oil, and any other nuts that you're not allergic to. You'll find some tips for doing this in chapter 14.

If you're the parent of a child with peanut allergies, you may have been lulled into a false sense of security by a widely reported study suggesting that as many as 20 percent of patients may outgrow their allergies. Even the study's author, pediatrician Robert Wood, M.D., associate professor of pediatrics at the Johns Hopkins University School of Medicine in Baltimore, urges parents not to reintroduce peanuts to allergic children unless it is done under a physician's supervision. *It is not a do-it-yourself experiment.*

> **DID YOU KNOW . . .**
>
> The oldest operating manufacturer and seller of peanut butter, Krema Products Company of Columbus, Ohio, has been selling peanut butter since 1908.
>
> SOURCE: THE NATIONAL PEANUT BOARD

In Dr. Wood's study, 220 children with peanut allergies were given a blood test, called RAST, that measured their levels of allergic antibodies to peanuts. "If their levels were below a certain point, we offered to give them a peanut challenge test," Dr. Wood explains. "They'd eat a certain dose of peanuts, and we'd observe them closely and treat them if they had a reaction."

As it turned out, the majority of the children had antibody levels too high to even be considered for a peanut challenge. But about 20 percent of the children had levels that showed they had outgrown their allergies.

"We are still treating peanut allergy as the most serious of all food allergies," Dr. Wood emphasizes. But he believes that reevaluating allergic children with the RAST test and the peanut challenge is worthwhile. "These fam-

---

KIDS AND PEANUT BUTTER DON'T ALWAYS MIX

As much as kids love peanut butter, the Peanut Butter Diet was designed with grownups in mind. If your child has a weight problem or other condition for which this diet might be helpful, be sure to check with your pediatrician before trying it.

In fact, some kids are just too young to eat peanut butter. Experts generally advise against giving peanut butter in the following situations.

Children under age 1. Before their first birthdays, kids are still learning to coordinate chewing and swallowing. The texture of peanut butter poses a risk because of the possibility of choking. By 18 months, however, nearly all children are developmentally ready to eat peanut butter. Just use common sense: Spread small, thin amounts on bread instead of giving it in large globs. As mentioned in chapter 1, Henry Heimlich, M.D., creator of the Heimlich Maneuver and president of the Heimlich Institute at Deaconess Hospital in Cincinnati, advises that no one, including adults, should eat peanut butter right off the spoon.

Children under age 3 who have a family history of allergies. If you or your spouse has a history of allergies, you shouldn't give peanut butter until after your child's third birthday, says Anne Munoz-Furlong, founder of the Food Allergy and Anaphylaxis Network in Fairfax, Virginia. Even if the parent's allergy is to another food or to pollen, the child would be considered high-risk. "We're hoping that by age 3, the immune system has matured enough that it won't recognize a harmless food like peanuts as harmful and create an allergy to it," Munoz-Furlong says.

ilies live day to day with the fear that their children are going to die from allergic reactions," he says. "Peanut allergies have a huge impact on life that can be completely removed once a child passes the peanut challenge."

You have difficulty swallowing. Older adults and people who have had strokes sometimes develop swallowing problems. Those who do may need to be evaluated by a speech and swallowing therapist. Depending on the nature of the problem, the therapist can make some very specific recommendations about foods and food consistencies that should be avoided.

You have extremely high triglycerides. As mentioned earlier, a diet high in monounsaturated fat from foods like peanut butter can help lower moderately elevated triglycerides. But according to the American Diabetes Association, if triglyceride levels reach or exceed 1,000 milligrams per deciliter (mg/dL) of blood, all dietary fat should be greatly reduced to protect against pancreatitis, or an inflamed pancreas. People with triglycerides this high should stick with an ultra low fat diet, getting no more than 10 percent of their total calories from fat. Since peanut butter is high in fat, even though it's the healthy monounsaturated kind, eliminating it makes sense. In addition, doctors can prescribe medication to help lower the risk of pancreatitis.

You're a woman who's pregnant, and you have a history of allergies. Studies are not conclusive about the relationship between pregnancy and a baby's sensitization to peanut butter. Still, because a peanut allergy can be a severe, lifelong condition, women with a history of allergies should restrict their consumption of peanut butter while they're expecting, advises Anne Munoz-Furlong, founder of the Food Allergy and Anaphylaxis Network in Fairfax, Virginia. For women who've been allergy-free, whether they eat peanut butter during pregnancy is their choice, Munoz-Furlong adds. Still, if you are pregnant, it's a good idea to consult your obstetrician before making any changes in your prenatal diet.

You're a woman who's breastfeeding, and you have a history of allergies. A study published in the April 2001 *Journal of the American Medical Association* reported that peanut protein consumed by a breastfeeding mother can pass into her breast milk, inadvertently exposing her baby. The authors of the study advised women with a history of allergies to avoid peanut-containing products while they're nursing.

PROCEED WITH CAUTION

While some people should avoid peanut butter altogether, others just need to watch their intakes. Here are some reasons to be cautious about your peanut butter consumption.

You have a history of kidney stones. People prone to kidney stones made from calcium oxalate may be advised by their doctors to cut back on certain foods, including peanut butter. If you've never passed a kidney stone that was saved and analyzed, you may not know whether your stones are of the calcium oxalate type. For you, avoiding peanut butter could be the safest—and least painful—course of action.

Still, the National Kidney and Urologic Diseases In-

THE AFLATOXIN MYTH

Have you read or heard that peanut butter can give you liver cancer? If so, you've been exposed to the aflatoxin myth, a misunderstanding that has created a fear of peanut butter in too many Americans.

Aflatoxin is a substance produced by a mold (field fungus) found in tropical and subtropical areas of the world, such as the southern United States. It often infects peanuts, wheat, corn, rice, and soybeans in those areas. If ingested in high amounts, it is believed to increase the risk of liver cancer. In developing countries, where food routinely spoils and becomes moldy, levels of aflatoxin may be quite high, and rates of liver cancer are far higher in regions of Asia and Africa than they are here.

"In the United States, eating 4 to 6 tablespoons of peanut butter 7 days a week, 365 days a year, shouldn't raise concern about aflatoxin," says food scientist Manfred Kroger, Ph.D., professor emeritus at Pennsylvania State University in University Park. That's because safety standards were put in place after the potential danger of aflatoxin was recognized in the 1970s.

Gillian Ann Zeldin, M.D., who specializes in liver transplant medicine at the University of Pennsylvania in Philadelphia, agrees. "Aflatoxin is a huge issue in some parts of the Third World," she says. "But in the United States, 4 to 6 tablespoons of peanut butter a day is not going to be harmful."

To safeguard Americans against aflatoxin-induced liver cancer, the FDA has set an acceptable aflatoxin level of no more than 20 parts per billion (ppb) for peanuts grown in the United States. Because of that regulation, peanuts are tested at many points, and any that exceed the cutoff are rejected.

According to the American Peanut Council, a trade organization, peanuts are tested for aflatoxin when they're delivered from the farmer to the sheller, then again when they leave the sheller. If they go to a warehouse, they're tested a third time before they're shipped out. They're tested a fourth time when they arrive at peanut butter manufacturers, which also test their finished products. And the FDA does shelf-testing of peanut butters.

If you're like me, though, you're thinking, "That's what they say they do. But do they really do it?" To satisfy our curiosity, my *Pre-*

vention colleagues and I sent 10 jars of peanut butter—all popular name brands and store brands—for testing at Trilogy Analytical Laboratory in Washington, Missouri. The results? Every brand came in well below the 20 ppb cutoff set by the FDA. Several brands had no detectable aflatoxin at all.

According to Bruce Malone, vice president of technical services for Trilogy, "Peanuts are probably the most analyzed product for aflatoxin. Eating 4 to 6 tablespoons of peanut butter a day is not going to be an issue."

One indication that our peanut butter products are safe seems to be the rate of liver cancer in the United States. It accounts for only 1.5 percent of all cancer cases, despite all the peanut butter we eat. For Americans, far more likely causes of liver cancer are hepatitis B and C and cirrhosis of the liver caused by alcohol abuse, according to the National Cancer Institute.

Commercial peanut butter is routinely checked and is safe, Dr. Kroger concludes. "In the average human diet, we'd have to eat ½ pound of highly contaminated peanut butter every day in order to be affected by aflatoxin," he says. "And we don't consume moldy food in general, because it is unsightly and tastes bitter. We reject it outright."

Ironically, the peanut butter that you may think is the healthiest may have more aflatoxin. "If you live in Georgia, for example, you may harvest your own peanuts," Dr. Kroger says. "If you happen to have an awfully moldy crop, and you work the peanuts into some homemade peanut butter and regularly eat large amounts of it, you may develop aflatoxicosis, or liver poisoning, after several months or years."

The moral of the story? Buy peanut butter at the supermarket. It's safe.

formation Clearinghouse recommends talking to your doctor before giving up any foods. In most cases, even potential troublemakers can be eaten in limited amounts.

You have gout. Gout is a painful disease caused by uric acid crystals being deposited in connective tissue or spaces in joints instead of passing from the body. The uric acid results from the breakdown of substances called purines, which come from certain foods. In the past, elimination of high-purine foods such as liver, sweetbreads, anchovies, and sardines has been a standard component of gout treatment.

These days, gout is managed with medications, including colchicine and nonsteroidal anti-inflammatory drugs. "At a practical level, people with gout can eat almost anything they want, with the exception of foods like sardines and anchovies," says John Klippel, M.D., medical director of the Arthritis Foundation in Washington, D.C. (Gout is considered part of the spectrum of joint diseases.) "In discussing diet with my patients, I've never once mentioned peanut butter." Still, just to be cautious, he advises patients with gout to consult their doctors before trying the 4 to 6 tablespoons of peanut butter a day that the Peanut Butter Diet recommends.

PART II

More Good Reasons
to Eat Peanut Butter

CHAPTER FOUR

Keep Your Heart Healthy

If you believe that the "expert-approved" way to a healthy heart is a low-fat diet, you're due for a very pleasant attitude adjustment. The U.S. government has just geared up its war on high cholesterol, but thanks to new research, you may not need to enlist in the low-fat diet army.

Updated guidelines, issued in May 2001 by the National Cholesterol Education Program (NCEP) of the National Institutes of Health, make the message clear: To stop unnecessary heart attack deaths, we need to make several changes in the way we treat and prevent heart disease. Many of these changes are embodied in the Peanut Butter Diet.

Besides advocating that more Americans be prescribed cholesterol-lowering medications, the revised NCEP guidelines include the following recommendations.

- Raising the level at which good HDL cholesterol—the kind that helps remove bad LDL cholesterol from the blood—is considered too low. The cutoff point used to be 35 milligrams per deciliter (mg/dL) of blood. Under the new guidelines, HDL should be at least 40 mg/dL. Studies show that diets rich in peanut butter do not reduce HDL, as low-fat diets sometimes do.
- Putting more emphasis on reducing high and even borderline-high triglycerides, a measure of total

fat present in the blood and a largely overlooked risk factor for heart attack—that is, until now. Research suggests that a rise in triglycerides of 88 mg/dL is associated with a 14 percent increase in heart disease risk in men and a whopping 37 percent increase in women. The American Heart Association defines normal triglycerides as less than 200 mg/dL, but some experts recommend staying below 120 mg/dL if you haven't had heart problems and below 90 if you have. Studies show that diets rich in peanut butter help reduce triglycerides.

- Paying more attention to a cluster of symptoms known as Syndrome X, or metabolic syndrome, which can dramatically raise heart attack risk even when total cholesterol levels appear normal. The Peanut Butter Diet fits the nutrition prescription for combating Syndrome X (as you'll see in chapter 6).

- Adopting an eating plan that limits saturated fat (the artery-clogging kind) to less than 7 percent of calories a day in order to reduce high cholesterol. The NCEP guidelines also allow up to 35 percent of daily calories from total fat, compared with their previous cap of 25 percent. The only

---

THE NATIONAL INSTITUTES OF HEALTH AGREES

In updating its dietary guidelines, the National Cholesterol Education Program (NCEP) of the National Institutes of Health made a dramatic change in the maximum amount of fat it recommends. The old guidelines allowed for 25 percent of calories from fat. As of May 2001, that "cap" rose to 35 percent of calories. The only caveat is that most of the fat be unsaturated—like the monounsaturated fat in peanut butter.

caveat is that most of that fat be unsaturated. Once again, the Peanut Butter Diet fits the bill perfectly.

WHY YOU WANT THOSE ARTERIES CLEAR

Let peanut butter help you keep your cholesterol profile in shape, so your blood vessels stay wide open instead of clogging with plaque. Stretched end to end, the vessels of your circulatory system, including the tiniest capillaries, would measure 60,000 miles. In one year, your heart beats 3 million times, and with each beat, it delivers oxygen and nutrients through your blood vessels to 300 trillion cells, including the cells that keep your heart beating. So do what you can to make sure that vital highway stays open!

RETHINKING THE LOW-FAT LAW

If the updated NCEP guidelines seem to contradict the nutritional advice that's been handed out for years, please keep in mind that nutritional science is a relatively young and continuously evolving field. Only within the past 20 or so years have scientists been able to look inside the body's cells to understand what's happening at the submicroscopic level with atoms and molecules. As advances in technology enable us to peer deeper into the body, and as we get an ever clearer picture of the effects of various foods, our prescriptions for the healthiest diet are bound to change.

For years, scientists believed that artery-clogging deposits of cholesterol were related purely to high intakes of fat. But that observation was made mainly in countries like our own, where much of the dietary fat was the saturated kind, from beef, butter, and cheese. The nutritional prescription for a healthy heart was based on cutting out as much fat as possible. Get down to 30 percent of calo-

ries from fat, or 25 percent, or, in the case of the Ornish
and Pritikin diets, 10 to 15 percent.

But back in the 1950s, a forward-thinking American
nutrition researcher named Ancel Keys, Ph.D., noticed
that in countries around the rim of the Mediterranean Sea,
cholesterol levels were low and heart attack deaths were
not as common as in the United States. Interestingly, the
traditional diets of these countries derived as much as 40
percent of their calories from fat.

What made these diets different, as Dr. Keys and other
researchers discovered, is that most of that fat comes
from olive oil, which is primarily monounsaturated fat. In
Crete, some farmers even
drink olive oil for breakfast!
It began to look as though
not all fat was bad—and in
fact, some of it might be
good.

> **DID YOU KNOW . . .**
>
> Women and children prefer
> creamy peanut butter, while
> most men opt for chunky.
>
> SOURCE: THE NATIONAL
> PEANUT BOARD

But proving that diets
rich in monounsaturated fat do not raise cholesterol required controlled, clinical studies—laboratory trials comparing cholesterol levels among groups of people eating
high-monounsaturated-fat diets, high-saturated-fat diets,
and every variation in between. Many of these studies
have now been done, most using olive oil as the source of
monounsaturated fat.

Their conclusion is beyond dispute. Yes, low-fat diets
reduce bad LDL cholesterol. But in some people, they
also decrease good HDL cholesterol and raise triglycerides, especially if the saturated fat is replaced with refined carbohydrates that are low in dietary fiber, like
white bread, bagels, and pretzels (which is what many
low-fat dieters do). On the other hand, the higher-fat
Mediterranean diet, rich in monounsaturated fat from

olive oil, lowers both bad LDL and triglycerides—without decreasing the good HDL.

ARGININE: A NEW ALLY FOR YOUR HEART

Scientists suspect that monounsaturated fat isn't solely responsible for peanut butter's potential heart benefits. High levels of fiber, folate, vitamin E, magnesium, and potassium, plus beta-sitosterol and resveratrol, undoubtedly play important roles.

But peanut butter has another secret ingredient that has yet to be mentioned: arginine, a component of peanut butter's protein.

Arginine is an amino acid that's found in relatively high concentrations in peanuts and nuts. Inside the body, it's used to manufacture nitric oxide, a once-ignored substance that heart experts now realize is crucial to heart health. With enough nitric oxide, the cells lining the inner layer of blood vessels are able to relax, allowing the vessels to dilate. That's important when a part of your body requires more blood, such as your heart whenever you climb the stairs.

Studies involving arginine supplements suggest that the amino acid may have a positive effect in patients with existing heart disease. The more arginine, the theory goes, the more nitric oxide. And the more nitric oxide, the more blood vessels can expand when they need to.

The amount of arginine in the average diet is well below the high levels of the amino acid used in studies. Nevertheless, several large dietary surveys have linked a high consumption of nuts with a significantly lower risk of heart disease. Nutrition experts now believe that arginine is part of the reason your heart loves nuts so much.

THE PROOF IS IN THE PEANUT BUTTER

All this is great news if you happen to love olive oil. But many Americans know next to nothing about olive oil or what to do with it. That's why researchers like Penny

Kris-Etherton, R.D., Ph.D., of Pennsylvania State University in University Park, began searching for other sources of monounsaturated fat that Americans could easily—and willingly—incorporate into their meals. Even though peanut butter is high in monounsaturated fat, the researchers needed to prove that olive oil didn't contain some special substance that was responsible for its wonderful effect on cholesterol levels.

In 1999, Dr. Kris-Etherton published a landmark study comparing diets with equal numbers of calories but various sources and levels of fat. Her research included the following diets:

- The typical American diet: 11 percent monounsaturated fat, 16 percent saturated fat, and 34 percent total fat
- The Step II diet, then recommended by the NCEP: 12 percent monounsaturated fat, 7 percent saturated fat, and 25 percent total fat
- An olive oil diet: 21 percent monounsaturated fat, 7 percent saturated fat, and 34 percent total fat
- A peanut oil diet: 17 percent monounsaturated fat, 7 percent saturated fat, and 34 percent total fat
- A peanut and peanut butter diet: 18 percent monounsaturated fat, 8 percent saturated fat, and 36 percent total fat

For her research, Dr. Kris-Etherton recruited 22 volunteers, all with cholesterol levels considered normal. The participants followed each diet for 24 days, with short breaks in between. All of the meals were prepared at Penn State's Metabolic Diet Study Center.

At the end of the study, Dr. Kris-Etherton compared the diets in terms of their effects on cholesterol and triglycerides. Both the Step II diet and all of the high-monounsaturated-fat diets reduced total cholesterol by 10 percent and bad LDL cholesterol by 14 percent. Good so far. But look what happened to triglycerides: On the low-fat Step II diet, they rose by 11 percent; on the high-mono diets, they dropped by 13 percent. The Step II diet also decreased good HDL cholesterol by 4 percent. On the high-mono diets, HDL stayed pretty much the same.

Based on the changes in cholesterol and triglyceride levels, the Step II diet appears to lower heart disease risk by an estimated 12 percent. In contrast, the peanut and peanut butter diet appears to lower heart disease risk by an estimated 21 percent—almost twice as much. These numbers are theoretical, but they show the heart-saving potential of this type of eating plan.

"Now there's evidence that a high-monounsaturated-fat diet may be preferable to a low-fat diet for cutting heart disease risk," Dr. Kris-Etherton says. "The evidence also shows that we can use peanuts and peanut products in designing a healthy high-monounsaturated-fat diet. That's good, because these foods fit in with typical American eating patterns and don't require drastic dietary changes."

PEANUT BUTTER SPREADS MONOS THICKEST

Compared with other popular spreads, peanut butter is the hands-down favorite for monounsaturated fat content.

FOOD	PORTION	MONOUNSATURATED FAT (G)	POLYUNSATURATED FAT (G)	SATURATED FAT (G)	CALORIES
Peanut Butter	2 Tbsp	8.0	4.4	3.3	190
Butter	2 Tbsp	7.2	1.2	15.0	216
Mayonnaise	2 Tbsp	6.4	11.6	3.4	200
Soy-nut butter	2 Tbsp	3.0	6.4	2.0	174
Cream cheese	2 Tbsp	2.8	0.4	2.8	98

MOUNTING EVIDENCE FOR MONOUNSATURATES

Dr. Kris-Etherton is by no means the only scientist who's looking at the positive effects of monounsaturated fat on heart disease risk. Based on data from a long-term study involving more than 80,000 nurses, Harvard researchers estimate that by replacing just 5 percent of calories from saturated fat with calories from unsaturated fat (which includes the monounsaturated kind in peanut butter), a woman could cut her heart disease risk by almost half.

As we've seen, a diet high in monounsaturated fat helps reduce triglycerides without lowering good HDL the way a standard low-fat diet can. To assess the health consequences of high triglycerides and low HDL, researchers in Denmark tracked men with known heart disease risk factors such as high LDL cholesterol, high blood pressure, low levels of physical activity, and cigarette use. The researchers found that over the course of 8 years, men with high triglycerides and low HDL were 35 percent more likely to have heart attacks than men with low triglycerides and high HDL, even though their other risk factors were the same. Clearly, a diet rich in monounsaturated fat, which cuts triglycerides without lowering HDL, can be good for your heart.

> **DID YOU KNOW . . .**
>
> Folks on the East Coast prefer creamy peanut butter, while those on the West Coast like the crunchy style.
>
> SOURCE: THE NATIONAL PEANUT BOARD

Of course, by slimming on the Peanut Butter Diet, you'll be controlling another major heart disease risk factor: overweight. And in chapter 5, you'll see how the

Peanut Butter Diet may help manage or prevent Type 2 (non-insulin-dependent) diabetes, now recognized as a major contributor to heart disease.

REVENGE OF THE NUT EATERS

If you're like me, you've been steering clear of peanuts and nuts as part of your effort to reduce your total fat intake. (Technically, peanuts are members of the legume family, but nutritionists tend to lump them in with tree nuts, like almonds and walnuts, because they have very similar nutritional profiles.)

Fortunately, a few stalwart folks have continued to eat nuts. And scientists are noticing something amazing about these people: They not only seem less prone to heart disease, they also appear to live longer.

In a 6-year study of more than 26,000 Seventh Day Adventists—who routinely eat healthy, plant-based diets—researchers at Loma Linda University in California found that those who ate moderate amounts of nuts at least five times a week were half as likely to experience heart attacks and coronary death as those who rarely ate nuts. Interestingly, the nut eaters were also significantly thinner than the rest of the group. This doesn't mean that nuts will make you thinner, but it does suggest they won't necessarily make you fat.

Another study tracked 34,000 women, all Iowa residents, over the course of 5 years. After adjusting for other risk factors such as smoking, obesity, and family history, the researchers concluded that the women who ate nuts were 40 percent less likely to die from heart disease than the women avoided them.

CHAPTER FIVE

Balance Blood Sugar
and Control Diabetes

Not so long ago, Type 2 diabetes was considered a disease that affected only those middle-aged and older. No longer. In the past 8 years, the incidence of Type 2—also known as non-insulin-dependent diabetes—has skyrocketed by 70 percent among people in their thirties.

Type 2 is even being diagnosed in teenagers and children. It accounts for up to 45 percent of all new diabetes cases in youngsters. Currently, an estimated 14.5 million Americans have the disease.

In Type 2 diabetes, your pancreas continues to produce insulin, the hormone that normally allows blood sugar to be absorbed by your cells and converted to energy. But for reasons not yet understood, your cells become resistant to the insulin you make. As a result, your blood sugar level rises. So does your insulin level, as your body tries even harder to get that blood sugar into your cells.

The higher your blood sugar and insulin rise over time, the more vulnerable you become to some very dire complications, including blindness, kidney failure, heart attack, and limb amputation. That's why the fact that diabetes is cropping up in children and teens is especially disconcerting. "The younger you are when you get diabetes, the tougher it is to avoid serious complications," explains Michael Engelgau, M.D., a diabetes researcher for the Centers for Disease Control and Prevention in Atlanta.

Experts pin the rise in Type 2 diabetes on two culprits:

our mushrooming obesity and our sedentary lifestyles. Simply put, we eat too many potato chips and rely on too many computer chips.

If you weigh more than you should, how do those extra pounds affect your chances of developing diabetes? Consider this: Among people with diabetes, about 90 percent are overweight. In one study of men who graduated from Johns Hopkins University Medical School, researchers determined that those who were overweight at age 25 were almost four times more likely to develop diabetes after age 50 than those who were not overweight at age 25.

This unhealthy union of overweight and diabetes—and the national health crisis that's brewing because of it—has experts so concerned that some are using a new term, *diabesity*, to describe it.

FIGHTING ON THREE FRONTS

Can the Peanut Butter Diet really help control diabetes? Absolutely—provided you follow it faithfully so that you shed those extra pounds. After all, while losing weight is one of the best ways to treat diabetes, gaining weight will only worsen the disease. And if you eat more peanut butter than is provided for in the menu plans, you will get heavier.

"Many of my overweight patients cannot have peanut butter in the house," reports Anne Daly, R.D., C.D.E. (certified diabetes educator), president of health care and education for the American Diabetes Association. "They are the people who unscrew the lid and get out the spoon whenever they're feeling stressed. I would not suggest peanut butter as their source of monounsaturated fat because I understand what they're going to do with it."

If this describes you and you have diabetes, I empha-

ARE YOU AT RISK FOR DIABETES?

Everyone age 45 and older should have a fasting plasma glucose test, which assesses blood sugar levels after an 8- to-12-hour fast. High numbers show that blood sugar isn't entering the body's cells, which is a sign of insulin resistance or an insulin shortfall. Readings above 126 milligrams per deciliter (mg/dL) of blood on two different days indicate diabetes. A reading above 110 mg/dL can signal impaired fasting glucose, a condition that can lead to Type 2 diabetes.

If your blood sugar levels are normal, they should be rechecked every 3 years. Get tested sooner—once a year—if any of the following situations apply to you.

- Your blood sugar is above 110
- You have a parent or sibling with diabetes
- You're overweight, particularly if you have "tummy fat" instead of hip fat
- You're physically inactive
- Your HDL cholesterol is below 35 mg/dL
- Your triglycerides are above 250 mg/dL
- You're African-American, Hispanic, Asian-American, or Native American
- You've ever been diagnosed with gestational diabetes or have given birth to more than one baby weighing over 9 pounds

---

size that the Peanut Butter Diet is not for you. You're at risk of eating too much peanut butter, and if you do, you could pack on pounds—*fast*. That would make me feel terrible. You wouldn't feel good, either.

On the other hand, if you have diabetes and you're able to stick with the calorie-controlled menu plans, you may benefit in three ways.

You'll Lose Weight
For some people, just slimming down, usually through a combination of diet and exercise, can be enough to return

blood sugar to normal levels. Still, you need to stay in touch with your physician so he can monitor your progress. If you're already taking diabetes medication and you lose some weight, your doctor may decide that you can reduce your dosage.

What worries physicians and dietitians about recommending a diet higher in fat to patients with diabetes—even if it's the healthy monounsaturated kind found in peanut butter—is that eating more fat can all too easily turn into eating more calories. That's because a gram of fat contains more than twice the calories of a gram of carbohydrates.

I understand their concerns. Frankly, unless you're knowledgeable about nutrition, incorporating more high-fat foods into your daily meals without increasing calories can be a challenge. That's one of the reasons we created the Peanut Butter Diet. We wanted to do all of the calculations for you—of total grams of fat; grams of monounsaturated and saturated fat, carbohydrate, and protein; and calories. That way, you wind up with menu plans high enough in monounsaturated fat to reap the health benefits but low enough in calories to lose weight. Plus, we wanted to make sure our diet is balanced with lots of fruits, vegetables, whole grains, and beans, and that it's rich in bone-building calcium.

> **DID YOU KNOW . . .**
>
> Each year, one-third to one-half of the U.S. peanut crop is used to make peanut butter.
>
> SOURCE: THE NATIONAL PEANUT BOARD

In one study mentioned in chapter 2, more people were able to slim down and stay slim on a higher-fat diet that included peanut butter than on a low-fat, high-carbohydrate diet. Presumably, that's because they enjoyed the higher-fat diet more.

If you've been diagnosed with diabetes, hopefully your doctor has advised you to see a registered dietitian, who can help you adjust your eating habits to control your blood sugar and shed extra pounds. This sort of professional guidance is especially important if you're thinking about switching from the low-fat, high-carbohydrate diet that's usually recommended for diabetes to a diet higher in monounsaturated fat. The Peanut Butter Diet can work for you, but rather than "winging it" on your own, *please* let a registered dietitian show you what to do. Ask your doctor for a recommendation or call the American Dietetic Association at (800) 366–1655 for names of dietitians in your area.

You'll Lower Your Triglycerides

Many people with diabetes also have high triglycerides and low levels of good HDL cholesterol. While the American Diabetes Association advocates a low-fat, high-carbohydrate diet as most effective for weight loss, the organization acknowledges that this sort of diet can actually backfire for some people by raising triglycerides and lowering HDL. Both changes can drive a person's heart attack risk higher.

On the other hand, many studies have demonstrated that when some carbohydrates are replaced with monounsaturated fat while keeping the total number of calories constant, triglyceride levels fall and HDL does not. And that *decreases* heart attack risk.

One of the first studies to demonstrate that a diet higher in monounsaturated fat could be more beneficial than a high-carbohydrate diet in treating diabetes was conducted simultaneously at the University of Texas Southwestern Medical Center in Dallas, Stanford University, the University of Minnesota–Minneapolis, and the University of California, San Diego. The results of the

5½-month study, which involved 42 patients with Type 2 diabetes, appeared in the *Journal of the American Medical Association* back in 1994.

At the time, patients with diabetes were routinely advised to reduce the saturated fat in their diets by cutting back on foods like beef, butter, and cheese and replacing them with carbohydrates like pasta, bread, and pretzels. Limiting saturated fat intake was essential, because diets high in saturated fat are among the major causes of high LDL, the bad cholesterol. High LDL increases heart attack risk, which is already elevated in people with diabetes.

> **DID YOU KNOW ...**
>
> November is Peanut Butter Lovers Month.
>
> SOURCE: THE NATIONAL PEANUT BOARD

Half of the 42 people in the study began with a high-carbohydrate diet, and half ate a diet high in monounsaturated fat. Halfway through the study period, the groups switched diets.

At all four study sites, the researchers found similar LDL levels in the study participants, regardless of diet. According to the principal author, Abhimanyu Garg, M.D., professor of internal medicine at the University of Texas Southwestern Medical Center, what impressed the researchers most were the changes they saw in blood sugar, insulin, and triglycerides. The high-monounsaturated-fat diet appeared to reduce all three measures, compared with the low-fat, high-carbohydrate diet.

Dr. Garg's conclusion, supported by many subsequent studies, is that a diet high in monounsaturated fat may be the healthiest for people with Type 2 diabetes because it helps reduce their risk of long-term complications, particularly heart attacks. He also notes that this type of diet may be more palatable for some people.

But even Dr. Garg does not shy away from the question of calories. "The most important issue in planning a high-monounsaturated-fat diet is to not exceed the required energy intake," he says. Translation: Don't overdo the peanut butter!

Fortunately, there's something about peanut butter that seems to make many people, including me, feel full longer than other foods can. Baltimore-based dietitian Colleen Pierre, R.D., agrees. "When I tell my patients to stir some peanut butter into their morning oatmeal, they are amazed at the way it keeps them more satisfied than plain oatmeal—right up to lunchtime," she says. You just may find that it's easier than you think to stick with the portions in the Peanut Butter Diet and not go hog-wild on calories.

THE AMERICAN DIABETES ASSOCIATION AGREES

What does the American Diabetes Association think about high-monounsaturated-fat diets? The organization states that if obesity and weight loss are the primary concerns, a reduced-fat diet may be the easiest way for some people to slim down. But it also says that if high triglycerides are a problem, "one approach that may be tried is a moderate increase in monounsaturated fat intake, with less than 10 percent of calories from saturated fat, and a more moderate carbohydrate intake." That describes the Peanut Butter Diet perfectly!

You'll Rein In Blood Sugar and Insulin

In this country, we're just starting to hear about something called the glycemic index. But in Canada, England, Australia, and elsewhere, it's one of the standard tools used by people with diabetes to control their blood sugar levels. According to the glycemic index, peanuts are just wonderful. So by extension, peanut butter is just wonderful, too.

The glycemic index, called GI for short, was created in the early 1980s by University of Toronto researchers. It ranks carbohydrate-containing foods according to their effects on blood sugar levels after they're eaten. Each of these foods is assigned a number.

Foods with a GI below 55 cause only a little blip in your blood sugar. Two examples are oranges, with a GI of 43, and lentil soup, with a GI of 44. Peanuts come in at 14, one of the lowest GIs of all foods. By extension, peanut butter ranks super-low on the GI scale, too.

Foods with a GI between 55 and 70 raise blood sugar a little higher. These include raisins, with a GI of 64, and popcorn, with a GI of 55. Foods with a GI above 70 send blood sugar soaring. At this end of the scale are bagels, with a GI of 72, and pretzels, with a GI of 83.

As nutrition scientists are learning, eating large amounts of high-GI foods is not healthy. When your blood sugar levels spike, your insulin production shifts into overdrive, too. In moderation, insulin is a good-guy hormone, escorting blood sugar into cells. But in excess, it becomes a killer, contributing to heart disease by raising blood pressure and triglycerides while lowering HDL cholesterol.

So far, the research examining the effects of low-GI diets and high-GI diets on diabetes looks promising. A Swedish study involving people with Type 2 diabetes found that compared with a high-GI diet, four weeks on a low-GI diet lowered blood sugar and insulin by 30 percent.

Low-GI foods may even help prevent diabetes. In a 6-year study of male health professionals, the men eating the lowest-GI diets were 25 percent less likely to develop the disease.

Despite the apparent benefits of a low-GI diet, experts say that no one should eat only low-GI foods. Rather, they advise cutting back on high-GI foods and trying to include at least one low-GI food in each meal.

The Peanut Butter Diet is designed to limit high-GI foods while maximizing low-GI foods like fruits, vegetables, and beans. By including luscious peanut butter in at least two of your meals or snacks every day, you'll be getting a super-low-GI food that can help maintain your blood sugar and insulin within a safe range.

Incidentally, the Peanut Butter Diet also supplies a healthy dose of fiber, averaging 29 grams per day for women and 35 grams per day for men. Eating lots of fiber is a proven way of keeping blood sugar on an even keel as well as reducing cholesterol. The next chapter will show you how the Peanut Butter Diet can help you fight another threat to your heart: Syndrome X.

A SECRET APPETITE SUPPRESSOR

If you're trying to slim down, eating more foods with a low glycemic index (GI), like peanuts and peanut butter, may work to your advantage. Preliminary research suggests that high-GI diets filled with refined carbohydrates like white bread, doughnuts, and snack crackers may actually increase hunger. That's because the flood of insulin after a high-GI meal ultimately sends blood sugar levels lower than if you'd never eaten. And low blood sugar may trigger hunger signals, according to Susan Roberts, Ph.D., professor of nutrition at Tufts University in Medford, Massachusetts.

CHAPTER SIX

Stop a Hidden Epidemic: Syndrome X

If you've never heard of Syndrome X—and many people haven't—then you need to know three crucial points about the condition. First, it's silent; you may get it and not even know it. Second, it's dangerous to your heart, even if your cholesterol readings seem perfectly normal. Third, it can be stopped—and the Peanut Butter Diet may be just the right medicine for it.

Syndrome X remains something of a mystery, although it's getting more and more attention from mainstream medical experts. It begins with insulin resistance, when the cells in your body don't respond to insulin as they should. This sets the stage for a cluster of symptoms that can include high triglycerides, low HDL, high blood pressure, and elevated blood sugar, all of which sneak up on your heart and rough it up before you even know what hit you.

Researchers estimate that Syndrome X may be responsible for up to half of all heart attacks. What's more, this silent killer may affect as many as 25 percent of adults.

Part of the reason that so few people know about the condition or its consequences is that doctors often miss detecting it. Why? "Because most of the patients who have Syndrome X show normal or close-to-normal cholesterol levels, so their doctors think they're fine," explains prominent investigator Jean-Pierre Despres, Ph.D., director of the lipid research center at Laval University Hospital in Quebec.

Yet so serious is this health issue that in May 2001, the National Cholesterol Education Program (NCEP) of the National Institutes of Health issued new guidelines that call upon doctors to focus on diagnosing and treating Syndrome X, or metabolic syndrome, as it's also called. The NCEP's experts are right to sound the alarm. As Scott Grundy, M.D., director of the center for human nutrition at the University of Texas Southwestern Medical Center in Dallas confirms, "Metabolic syndrome has emerged as being a very strong contributor to early heart disease."

The good news is, if you are diagnosed with Syndrome X, you can take measures to treat it. They include adopting the delicious Peanut Butter Diet.

TROUBLE FROM THE START

The key player in Syndrome X is insulin, a hormone that's secreted by your pancreas into your bloodstream. Insulin's job is to escort blood sugar, or glucose, into your body's muscle and fat cells. Once inside these cells, glucose becomes the fuel that produces the energy to keep you alive and moving around.

When Syndrome X kicks in, insulin knocks on the doors of your cells, but they don't open up—at least not often enough. Sensing that undelivered glucose is floating around in your bloodstream, your pancreas releases more and more insulin into your blood. When levels of the hormone become chronically elevated, you've got trouble. In particular, your risk of heart attack soars.

Exactly why cells become resistant to insulin isn't clear. It seems to have some connection to being overweight—especially if you carry the extra pounds around your middle instead of on your hips and thighs (in other words, you have an apple shape instead of a pear shape).

Whatever the cause of insulin resistance, its effects are downright nasty. You may develop high triglycerides, now recognized as a major risk factor for heart disease. (If you're not familiar with them, triglycerides are the chemical form of fat.) Your HDL cholesterol, the kind that removes cholesterol from your bloodstream, goes down—another major risk factor for heart disease. But your total cholesterol and LDL cholesterol, the kind that forms plaques and clogs arteries, may remain normal. If your doctor looks at only those numbers, he may miss Syndrome X.

> **DID YOU KNOW . . .**
>
> Americans eat more than 700 million pounds of peanut butter each year.
>
> SOURCE: THE NATIONAL PEANUT BOARD

Worse, if your total cholesterol and LDL cholesterol are higher than they should be, your doctor may advise you to try a low-fat, high-carbohydrate diet. This can actually make Syndrome X worse instead of better. It's one of the most dangerous aspects of the condition.

Besides increasing triglycerides and decreasing HDL, Syndrome X can raise blood levels of fibrinogen, a substance that encourages your blood to clot spontaneously. This is dangerous because a blood clot that finds its way into a narrowed artery can trigger a heart attack or stroke. Just as ominous, Syndrome X can drive up levels of plasminogen activator inhibitor (PAI-1), leaving your body less able to naturally dissolve any clots that do develop.

Other symptoms characteristic of Syndrome X include high blood pressure and elevated blood sugar levels, both of which can raise your risk for a heart attack. You needn't have all of the symptoms to be diagnosed with the condition, however.

THREE SIGNS TO WATCH FOR

If you can answer yes to all of the following questions, consult your doctor. You may very well have Syndrome X.

- Does your waist measure more than 35 inches?
- Is your cholesterol ratio (total cholesterol divided by HDL cholesterol) more than 5?
- Are your triglycerides above 175 mg/dL?

ARE YOU AT RISK?

Since insulin resistance sets the stage for Syndrome X, testing for high levels of insulin would seem to be the most obvious means of diagnosis. Yet while the hormone plays an important role in the condition, it's extremely difficult to measure. The best test is complicated, expensive, and unpleasant, experts say. They're working on a more practical alternative, though. "I think that 4 or 5 years from now, people will know their insulin levels the way they know their cholesterol levels," says researcher George Howard, Ph.D., professor of biostatistics at the University of Alabama at Birmingham.

Of course, if you suspect that you have Syndrome X, you don't want to wait that long to get a definitive diagnosis, much less begin treatment. In your case, the following tests can help pinpoint the condition. Several require a doctor's intervention. (And if your doctor hasn't heard about Syndrome X, I suggest you give him a copy of this chapter to read.)

Measure your waist. As I mentioned earlier, the symptoms associated with Syndrome X seem most common in people who have excess abdominal fat. To find out whether you're packing too many pounds on your abdomen, simply measure your waist. That's right, measure your waist *only*. New research suggests that this number may be more accurate than the waist-to-hip ratio for assessing fat around the middle.

Dr. Despres's research has shown that for both women and men, a waistline larger than 35 inches usually indicates the presence of Syndrome X. For his part, Dr. Despres believes that abdominal fat may have the strongest correlation to the condition. That's why he refers to it as Big Belly Syndrome.

Calculate your cholesterol ratio. Another indicator of Syndrome X is a ratio of total cholesterol to HDL cholesterol that's above 5, Dr. Despres says. To determine your ratio, simply divide your total reading by your HDL reading. Don't know these numbers? Well, you should be having your cholesterol checked at least once every 5 years starting at age 20, and possibly more often if you're older or if you have other risk factors for heart disease.

When you do have your cholesterol checked, you'll also learn your LDL level. It, too, is an important measure of heart health. Just keep in mind that people with Syndrome X often have LDL numbers within a normal range.

Find out your triglyceride level. When you eat too many calories or drink too much alcohol, the excess turns into triglycerides. The American Heart Association defines a normal triglyceride reading as less than 200 milligrams per deciliter (mg/dL) of blood. But experts knowledgeable about Syndrome X say that people with triglycerides above 175 mg/dL and a waist measurement above 35 inches have an 80 percent chance of developing the condition. By comparison, those whose triglycerides are below 175 and whose waist measurements are below 35 inches have only a 10 percent chance of developing Syndrome X.

Keep tabs on your blood sugar. Several people with Syndrome X show increased levels of fasting blood sugar, which can be checked along with your cholesterol as part of a routine physical exam. A blood sugar reading above 100 mg/dL could point to Syndrome X, especially if the high reading is accompanied by high triglycerides, low HDL, and a big waist.

Know your blood pressure reading. Your doctor probably takes your blood pressure every time you visit his office. Your systolic pressure, the top number in your reading, should be under 130; your diastolic pressure, the bottom number, should be under 85. This is true for anyone, regardless of whether they have Syndrome X.

THE BEST RX: WEIGHT LOSS

If all of these tests suggest that you do have Syndrome X, the first—and most important—thing you can do is unload any extra pounds you may be carrying. It is well-known that losing weight helps reduce insulin resistance. Dr. Despres recommends that you slim down enough to get your waist measurement below 35 inches.

To do this, you *must* get active. Being sedentary not only packs on pounds, it also raises your risk for Syndrome X. But exercise can help control and even reverse the condition by perking up an important protein that enables insulin to transport blood sugar into muscle cells. Since these cells are the most voracious users of blood sugar, they are also the biggest employers of insulin. In effect, exercise defeats insulin resistance and overweight, two key players in Syndrome X, in one fell swoop. (For real-world advice on incorporating more physical activity into your daily routine, see chapter 15.)

That said, weight loss doesn't happen by exercise alone. You also need to curb your calorie intake—but following the standard low-fat, high-carbohydrate diet could be a serious mistake. Although this type of eating plan is very healthy for most people, it can actually worsen symptoms in those with Syndrome X. For them, eating lots of carbs can send triglycerides even higher and HDL even lower.

It's easy to see why. Carbohydrates—starches and sweets like white bread and doughnuts—are converted into blood sugar. The more blood sugar you have, the more insulin your pancreas manufactures. But since your cells won't let insulin do its job, you end up with even higher levels of the hormone after eating a high-carb meal. And as we've seen, one of the outcomes of elevated insulin is increased triglycerides and decreased HDL, both of which are very bad for your heart.

This is why getting a proper diagnosis for Syndrome X is so important. To slim down, most people instinctively switch to a low-fat, high-carbohydrate diet. They may even follow it religiously. All the while, they have no idea that they may be putting their hearts at even greater risk.

THE AMERICAN HEART ASSOCIATION AGREES

In its updated dietary guidelines, issued in 2000, the American Heart Association offers the following advice: "For individuals diagnosed with [Syndrome X], it may be desirable to avoid very low fat, high carbohydrate diets and to emphasize unsaturated fats...." The Peanut Butter Diet fills this prescription perfectly.

HOW THE PEANUT BUTTER DIET CAN HELP

For people with Syndrome X, the traditional low-fat, high-carbohydrate diet—with its breads, bagels, and pretzels—is out. This begs the question: Which diet is in?

For an answer, we need look no further than the Pennsylvania State University study discussed in detail in chapter 4. This study compared the effects of low-fat, high-carbohydrate diets with those of diets that were slightly lower in carbohydrates but higher in monounsaturated fat, including one particular eating plan that featured peanuts and peanut butter. (All were low in saturated fat, a must for any healthy weight-loss program.)

As you may remember, while both types of diets lowered total cholesterol and bad LDL cholesterol, only those higher in monounsaturated fat also reduced triglycerides. What's more, the low-fat, high-carbohydrate diet actually decreased good HDL cholesterol, something the diets higher in monounsaturated fat did not do.

In other words, a diet higher in monounsaturated fat helped overcome two major symptoms of Syndrome X: high triglycerides and low HDL, both of which imperil your heart. Because it's naturally rich in monounsaturated fat, the Peanut Butter Diet just may enable you to control or even reverse Syndrome X.

According to the American Heart Association, a diet higher in polyunsaturated fat—the kind found in corn oil and soybean oil—may work just as well. Which approach is better? So far, all researchers know is that both can help.

So if you're a fan of peanut butter—or nuts, avocados, or olive oil, all of which are excellent sources of monounsaturated fat—your choice may be clear. Just remember that if you try the Peanut Butter Diet, you must stick with the peanut butter portions recommended in the menu plans in chapters 11 and 12. Otherwise, you'll consume too many calories, which means you'll gain weight rather than lose it. And that can make Syndrome X even worse.

Diets high in monounsaturated fat, like the Peanut Butter Diet, work *only* when calorie intake is controlled. In fact, this is true of any eating plan intended for weight loss. Having preset menus to follow is one way to make sure that you don't unintentionally go calorie-crazy until you get the hang of higher-fat meals. That's why for the Peanut Butter Diet, my colleagues and I have created the menus and counted all the calories for you.

CHAPTER SEVEN

Stock Up on Scarce Nutrients

Do you know what is possibly the most unappreciated benefit of peanut butter? It's the only comfort food I know of that's literally stuffed with nutrients that you're likely to run low on—some often-overlooked nutrients such as folate, zinc, magnesium, potassium, and copper, as well as vitamin E. What's more, it's unusually high in resveratrol and beta-sitosterol, two intriguing natural compounds that scientists believe help fight cancer and heart disease. As if that weren't enough, it's also rich in fiber, a little-known weight-loss aid.

Many nutrition professionals are just becoming aware of peanut butter's nutrient-dense payload. Janis Jibrin, M.S., R.D., a dietitian and nutrition writer based in Washington, D.C., says that only while researching the 100 healthiest foods for women did she realize all that peanut butter has to offer. "I was already eating it every day," she notes. "Now that I know how amazingly healthy it is, I feel great about it." But she stresses that portion control is essential, just as I do.

By following the Peanut Butter Diet, you'll be stocking up on vitamins, minerals, and other compounds that your body may well need more of for maximum health. Let's look at some of these vital nutrients a bit more closely.

MAJOR NUTRITION IN EVERY MORSEL

If you eat peanut butter as directed in the daily menu plans (see chapters 11 and 12), you'll be getting 10 percent or more of the Daily Values (DVs) for the following vitamins and minerals.

Folate: Not Just for Moms-to-Be

Long overshadowed by its B vitamin brethren, folate has come into its own as a nutritional superstar. It has many potential benefits.

It supports the development of healthy babies. In the 1990s, several studies proved that if women of childbearing age were to consume at least 400 micrograms of folate a day before the time of conception, they'd be less than half as likely to give birth to babies with serious brain and spinal cord defects. That's because folate plays an essential role in helping the body make perfect copies of DNA, the cell's master plan for reproduction. Other research indicates that folic acid (the supplement form of folate) taken before conception may reduce the number

---

HOW THE SOURCES STACK UP: FOLATE

To get the roughly 47 micrograms of folate in 4 tablespoons of peanut butter, you'd need to eat one of the following:

5 raw carrots, each 7½ inches long
7 ounces of cooked trout
1¼ cups of cooked green beans
1½ cups of canned sweet potatoes
1½ cups of red raspberries

THE PEANUT BUTTER DIET PAYOFF

With just the nutrient-dense peanut butter that's the star ingredient in the Peanut Butter Diet, you'll help replenish your body's supply of these critical vitamins and minerals.

NUTRIENT	FUNCTION	WOMEN'S DIET (4 Tbsp)	% DAILY VALUE*	MEN'S DIET (6 Tbsp)	% DAILY VALUE*
Folate	Prevents birth defects; supports heart health	47.4 mcg	11.9	71 mcg	17.8
Vitamin E	Supports heart health, especially in people with diabetes; may fight mental decline	9.6 IU	31.8	14.3 IU	47.8
Zinc	Strengthens the immune system; helps preserve vision	1.8 mg	12	2.7 mg	18
Magnesium	Relaxes blood vessels, which helps lower blood pressure	100 mg	25	150 mg	37.5
Potassium	Fights high blood pressure and strokes	428 mg	12.2	642 mg	18.3
Copper	Strengthens the immune system	0.33 mg	16.5	0.5 mg	24.8

*The DV is a one-size-fits-all recommended intake for each nutrient, as established by the FDA. For some nutrients, the DVs differ somewhat from the Recommended Dietary Allowances (RDA) and Adequate Intakes (AI), which are periodically revised by the National Academies' Institute of Medicine.

of children born with heart defects. The B vitamin may even lower the risk of Down syndrome.

The trouble is, most women of childbearing age average only about 204 micrograms of folate a day. By eating the 4 tablespoons of peanut butter provided for them in the Peanut Butter Diet, however, they'll get an extra 47 micrograms a day. That's almost 12 percent of the recommended DV of 400 micrograms.

So crucial is folate for preventing birth defects that the U.S. Public Health Service advises all women of child-bearing age to eat folate-rich foods and, as insurance, to take 400 micrograms of folic acid in a multivitamin/mineral supplement.

It cuts your risk of heart attack. Researchers have determined that low levels of folate allow homocysteine, a natural by-product of the breakdown of amino acids in the body, to accumulate in the blood. Too much homocysteine can set the stage for heart disease by damaging arteries and prompting the buildup of plaque on artery walls. Getting more folate helps remove homocysteine from the blood. In fact, people with higher intakes of folate have both lower levels of homocysteine and lower risk of heart disease.

Incidentally, women aren't the only ones running low on folate. Among men, the average intake is 274 micrograms a day. They can get another 71 micrograms, nearly 18 percent of the DV, by eating the 6-tablespoon portion of peanut butter recommended for them in the Peanut Butter Diet.

It may protect against cancer and Alzheimer's disease. Diet surveys strongly suggest that people who consume more folate are less likely to develop colon and prostate cancer. Other research has linked higher blood levels of the B vitamin with a reduced risk of Alzheimer's disease.

Vitamin E: Extra Heart Protection

Few foods supply more than modest amounts of vitamin E, but peanut butter is one of the exceptions. By following the Peanut Butter Diet, you'll stock up on a nutrient that has some impressive health benefits. Here are a few examples.

It safeguards your heart. Some research has identified a connection between vitamin E and a reduced risk of heart disease. In one clinical study, the nutrient seemed to help protect against second heart attacks.

It prevents diabetes complications. Diabetes is considered a major risk factor for heart attack. Researchers are actively investigating vitamin E's potential to prevent the cardiovascular damage that's often associated with diabetes. People who have the disease are known to produce exceptionally high levels of unstable particles called free radicals, which ultimately contribute to clogged arteries. As an antioxidant, vitamin E can help neutralize those free radicals before they cause harm.

It may preserve mental function. Several diet surveys suggest that older people with higher vitamin E intakes perform better on memory skill tests. Researchers are eager to test whether keeping lots of vitamin E on board can actually help you stay sharp as you age.

While the DV of vitamin E is 30 IU, the average intake for women is just 9 IU, and for men, 12 IU. You may be getting even less if you're on a low-fat diet, since vitamin E is most abundant in foods that are high in fat. Peanut butter is high in fat, too—only it's the monounsaturated kind, which is healthier for you.

In the women's version of the Peanut Butter Diet, 4 tablespoons of peanut butter a day supplies 9.6 IU of vitamin E, almost 32 percent of the DV. The 6-tablespoon portion for men delivers 14.3 IU, almost 48 percent of the DV.

Because of studies indicating that extra vitamin E may be beneficial, *Prevention* magazine recommends that you also consider taking 100 to 400 IU of the nutrient in supplement form.

HOW THE SOURCES STACK UP: VITAMIN E

To get the almost 10 IU of vitamin E in 4 tablespoons of peanut butter, you'd need to eat one of the following:

　4 cups of cubed papaya
　4 cups of frozen blueberries
　20 fresh apricots
　20 pieces of whole wheat bread
　20 bananas

Zinc: A Versatile Mineral

Your body manufactures hundreds of chemical compounds to support its basic functions. Zinc needs to be present for more than 100 of them to work.

One of the mineral's critical roles is to support the production of compounds that tell your immune system what to do when bacteria and viruses attack. Adequate zinc is also important for preserving your eyesight. Too bad the average American woman gets only about 9 milligrams of zinc a day, compared with the DV of 15 milligrams. The average man fares a bit better, getting 13 milligrams a day.

Maintaining the zinc supply can be especially difficult for people who've cut back on red meat, one of the top sources of the mineral. For them, and for anyone concerned about their zinc intake, the Peanut Butter Diet may be a smart choice. The 4 tablespoons of peanut butter a day in the women's version of the diet provides 1.8 milligrams of zinc, or 12 percent of the DV. In the men's version, 6 tablespoons of peanut butter delivers 2.7 milligrams of zinc, or 18 percent of the DV.

You should be aware that a report from the National Academies' Institute of Medicine says that we may need less zinc than the DV calls for. If that's the case, the Peanut Butter Diet goes even further in fulfilling your body's zinc requirement.

HOW THE SOURCES STACK UP: ZINC

To get the 1.8 milligrams of zinc in 4 tablespoons of peanut butter, you'd need to eat one of the following:

1 cup of cooked lima beans
3 cooked whole artichokes
1½ cups of cooked brown rice
40 dried plums (prunes)
3 cups of cooked broccoli

Magnesium: Controls Blood Pressure

Most of your body's magnesium is found in your bones and teeth, where it helps keep these structures strong. Smaller but vital amounts of the mineral also circulate in your bloodstream, where it helps the muscles of your heart and blood vessels relax. This keeps your blood pressure from rising too high.

Why is this a very good thing? Because in high blood pressure, the force of blood cells beating and crashing against artery walls can inflame them and harden them, inviting plaque to build up and forcing your heart to work harder. Uncontrolled high blood pressure puts you at greater risk for heart attack, stroke, and mental decline as you grow older.

Unfortunately, the average woman gets only about 228

milligrams of magnesium a day, and the average man gets 302 milligrams. Both numbers fall well below the DV of 400 milligrams. But once again, peanut butter can come to the rescue. Four tablespoons gives women 100 milligrams of magnesium, or 25 percent of the DV. For men, 6 tablespoons provides 150 milligrams, or 37 percent of the DV.

HOW THE SOURCES STACK UP: MAGNESIUM

To get the 100 milligrams of magnesium in 4 tablespoons of peanut butter, you'd need to eat one of the following:

- 4 cups of cooked pasta
- 2½ cups of cooked beets
- 10 fresh pears
- 20 cooked eggs
- 4 cups of grape juice

Potassium: Another Heart Helper

This mineral proved its merit in the now-famous study called Dietary Approaches to Stop Hypertension, or DASH for short. Study participants who consumed foods rich in potassium—fruits and vegetables, low-fat dairy products, and nuts—saw their blood pressure drop considerably. In some cases, the reduction matched what

---

HOW THE SOURCES STACK UP: POTASSIUM

To get the 428 milligrams of potassium in 4 tablespoons of peanut butter, you'd need to eat one of the following:

- 3¼ cups of cooked oatmeal
- 2 cups of cottage cheese
- 10½ ounces of cooked chicken liver
- 1½ cups of blackberries
- 1¼ cups of pineapple juice

would have occurred if the person had been taking prescription blood pressure medication. In a separate study, just one serving a day of a potassium-rich food cut the risk of stroke by almost 40 percent.

The DV for potassium is 3,500 milligrams. By comparison, the average woman gets about 2,237 milligrams a day, and the average man, about 2,896 milligrams a day. Peanut butter can help make up for the shortfall. In the Peanut Butter Diet, the 4-tablespoon allowance for women supplies 428 milligrams of potassium, or about 12 percent of the DV. In 6 tablespoons, men get 642 milligrams, or more than 18 percent of the DV.

Copper: Just a Little Means a Lot

Experts say that a poor diet is the single biggest reason that the immune system breaks down. A poor diet runs low on key nutrients, and copper could be the weakest link. While the DV is 2 milligrams, women average 1.1 milligrams a day, and men, 1.5 milligrams. "Even a marginal copper deficiency suppresses immune function in laboratory animals and cultured human cells," says Mark Failla, Ph.D., chairman of the human nutrition department at Ohio State University in Columbus.

> **DID YOU KNOW . . .**
>
> Arachibutyrophobia (pronounced *i-ra-kid-bu-Tl-ro-pho-bi-a*) is the fear of peanut butter getting stuck to the roof of your mouth.
>
> SOURCE: THE NATIONAL PEANUT BOARD

And it's not just colds and flu that your immune system battles. Increasingly, scientists recognize that a strong immune system may be one of your best defenses against cancer.

Want to get more copper in a most delicious way? In the women's version of the Peanut Butter Diet, 4 tablespoons of peanut butter supplies 0.33 milligram, or 16.5 percent of the DV for this stay-well mineral. For men, 6

HOW THE SOURCES STACK UP: COPPER

To get the 0.33 milligram of copper in 4 tablespoons of peanut butter, you'd need to eat one of the following:

    1½ cups of cooked green peas
    3 cups of cooked white rice
    6 cups of apple juice
    3 cups of cooked red cabbage
    ¾ cup of raisins

---

tablespoons of peanut butter delivers almost 0.5 milligram, or close to 25 percent of the DV.

According to a report from the National Academies' Institute of Medicine, we may not need as much copper as the DV suggests. That means the Peanut Butter Diet covers an even greater proportion of our ideal daily intake.

EXCITING EXTRA INGREDIENTS

Nestled among all those vitamins and minerals in peanut butter are several other healing ingredients. Two of them, resveratrol and beta-sitosterol, are phytochemicals that scientists are studying as potential fighters of heart disease and cancer. Another is fiber, which has impressive benefits all its own.

Resveratrol: Stops Clots Cold

If you've already heard of resveratrol (res-VER-a-trol), it was probably in connection with red wine. Resveratrol is a naturally occurring compound that helps some plants fend off disease. It's concentrated in the skins of red grapes, which is why it turns up in red wine. Studies have linked moderate consumption of red wine (one glass a day for women, two for men) with lower rates of heart disease. Scientists attribute red wine's effects in part to resveratrol, which helps keep platelets in the blood from sticking together and forming clots, the immediate triggers of most heart attacks and strokes. Resveratrol may also help prevent bad LDL cholesterol from building plaque on artery walls.

While a 4-ounce glass of red wine contains about 640 micrograms of resveratrol, women who drink even one glass a day may raise their risk of breast cancer. Fortunately, they don't need red wine to get resveratrol. According to Timothy Sanders, Ph.D., a USDA Agricultural Research Service research leader and professor of food science at North Carolina State University in Raleigh, 4 tablespoons of peanut butter provides about 26 micrograms of resveratrol. In contrast, an entire quarter-pound of Concord grapes averages only 10 micrograms.

Resveratrol may help fight cancer, too. In animal studies at the University of Illinois at Chicago, the compound stopped the growth of cells with damaged DNA, which can be a precursor of cancer.

Beta-Sitosterol: Keeps Cholesterol in Check

You may be familiar with beta-sitosterol (BE-ta-si-TOS-terol) from advertisements for a cholesterol-lowering margarine called Take Control. Research shows that when consumed with food, beta-sitosterol blocks the absorption of cholesterol by the body. It also prevents the reabsorption of cholesterol that's transported from the liver into the intestines by bile. In studies, using Take Control as directed has lowered levels of bad LDL cholesterol by about 10 percent, while leaving good HDL cholesterol unaffected.

The beta-sitosterol that's an ingredient in the margarine is refined from soybeans. The good news is, peanut butter has its own natural supply of the compound!

How much beta-sitosterol do you need to improve your cholesterol profile? According to the FDA, "Foods containing at least 0.65 gram per serving of vegetable oil sterol esters [beta-sitosterol], eaten twice a day with meals for a total daily intake of at least 1.3 grams, as part of a diet low in saturated fat and cholesterol, may reduce the risk of heart disease." By consuming the 4 tablespoons of peanut butter recommended in the Peanut Butter Diet, a woman would get 0.1 gram of beta-sitosterol. That's not as much as the FDA recommends, but it probably contributes to the diet's cholesterol-lowering power.

For guys who adopt the Peanut Butter Diet, 6 tablespoons of peanut butter supplies 0.15 gram of beta-sitosterol. That's significant because recent research has revealed that consuming 0.12 gram of beta-sitosterol a day may help relieve the urinary urgency and frequency caused by benign prostatic hyperplasia (an enlarged prostate gland). It's interesting to note that saw palmetto extract, a widely recommended herbal remedy for prostate problems, contains phytosterols, the class of compounds that includes beta-sitosterol.

Finally, one of the world's top beta-sitosterol researchers, Atif Awad, R.D., Ph.D., associate professor and director of the nutrition program at the State University of New York at Buffalo, has conducted both test-tube and animal studies in which the compound appeared to inhibit the growth and spread of colon and breast cancers. In one of Dr. Awad's experiments, mice inoculated with human breast cancer cells and fed beta-sitosterol still developed tumors, but the growths were 33 percent smaller. In addition, the spread of cancer cells to the lymph nodes and lungs was 20 percent less. Dr. Awad notes that in Europe, beta-sitosterol is now being added to milk and other food products.

Fiber: Prevention in Every Gram

The average American woman gets about 12 grams of fiber a day. That's less than half of the 25 to 35 grams nutrition experts recommend. The average man consumes about 16 grams, which is slightly better, but still way too low.

Most people equate fiber with roughage, and peanut butter is anything but roughage. So you may be surprised to learn that 4 tablespoons of peanut butter, the daily allotment for women in the Peanut Butter Diet, supplies 4

CALORIES THAT DON'T COUNT

I'll bet the fiber in peanut butter has one benefit that will totally surprise and delight you: It seems to erase some of the calories you eat!

In one admittedly small study from the USDA Human Nutrition Research Center in Beltsville, Maryland, increasing daily fiber intake from 13 grams to 26 grams resulted in the absorption of 90 fewer calories. Apparently, all that fiber hangs on to some of the calories you consume and escorts them right out of your body before they can make their way into your bloodstream and onto your thighs. For every gram of fiber you add to your diet, you subtract roughly 7 calories.

Doesn't sound like much? Let's do the math. A woman who adopts the Peanut Butter Diet, with its fiber-rich peanut butter, fruits, vegetables, beans, and whole grains, will take in about 29 grams of fiber a day. That's an increase of about 17 grams, based on an average intake of 12 grams a day. If each extra gram of fiber prevents the absorption of 7 calories, this woman would absorb 43,435 fewer calories over the course of a year. Since 3,500 calories equals 1 pound, she could lose 12 pounds within a year simply by eating more fiber.

Men get about 35 grams of fiber a day on the Peanut Butter Diet, an increase of 19 over their average daily intake of 16 grams. Theoretically, a guy could take off 14 pounds in a year. A little extra fiber is all he needs.

grams of fiber. The 6 tablespoons recommended for men delivers 6 grams.

Dozens of studies have linked fiber-rich diets with a reduced risk of heart disease, stroke, diabetes, colon cancer, and breast cancer. I'm sure you've seen the headlines announcing that one study found no connection between fiber intake and colon cancer rates. But I can guarantee that if you were to assemble all of the relevant studies and look through them, you'd be pretty convinced that getting more fiber can make you healthier in many ways.

Is it the fiber itself? Is it other ingredients found in fiber-rich foods? Is it both? Scientists don't know for sure, but most are convinced that something about high-fiber diets is good for you. And now you know that peanut butter is a delicious way to get the fiber you need.

MORE FAT, MORE NUTRIENTS

Here are two little-known benefits of a diet that's higher in fat, such as the Peanut Butter Diet.

- You'll absorb more of the fat-soluble nutrients, which require fat to be digested and pass through the wall of your intestine. They include vitamins A, D, E, and K.
- You'll absorb more of the compounds from the carotenoid family, such as the beta-carotene in carrots (a potential breast cancer fighter) and the lycopene in tomatoes (a likely prostate cancer foe).

PART III

How to Do the
Peanut Butter Diet

CHAPTER EIGHT

Take the Ping-Pong Pledge

Raise your right hand and repeat after me: "When I follow the Peanut Butter Diet, I solemnly promise to stick with the recommended portion size. If I cheat and eat more peanut butter than that, I know I will gain weight—*fast*."

I hope that got your attention. Just in case you've missed the point before, the very tricky part of following a diet with more fat—even the healthy monounsaturated fat in peanut butter—is that you can easily take in too many calories unless you're religious about portion control.

Every single expert I interviewed for this book empha-

HOW TO HANDLE TRIGGER FOODS

At luxurious Canyon Ranch Health Resort in Tucson, nutritionist Jim Glaser, R.D., has counseled thousands of guests about healthy weight loss. One topic that comes up often is trigger foods—foods that people just can't seem to stop eating once they start.

Glaser's advice on how to deal with these temptations may be surprising. "Whether it's peanut butter or chocolate or bread or whatever, I recommend that it be built into a person's diet on a regular basis," he explains. "This helps to prevent bingeing on that food. It lessens the trigger ability of the food."

Glaser recognizes that for some people, trigger foods pose a real challenge. "But ultimately," he says, "you have to know how to manage your trigger foods if you want to maintain your weight loss for the long term."

sized the potential danger of ballooning calorie intake if
people simply add peanut butter to their existing diets or
if they don't take responsibility for measuring the amount
of peanut butter they're eating. "Calories track with fat,"
says nutrition authority Penny Kris-Etherton, R.D.,
Ph.D., of Pennsylvania State University in University
Park. "If you want a higher-fat diet that includes peanut
butter, you've got to stick with the program."

GENEROUS PORTIONS ALLOWED

Don't worry, though. The Peanut Butter Diet allows sur-
prisingly ample portions of peanut butter. Women get two
servings a day of 2 tablespoons each; men get three servings a day of 2 tablespoons each. That's a nice, satisfying
glob of peanut butter. It's not as though you're being
teased with teensy portions, like a teaspoon a day. That
couldn't possibly satisfy anyone's cravings.

That said, because each 2-tablespoon serving contains
190 calories, you're virtually certain to pack on pounds if
you eat more peanut butter than the diet provides. You'll
feel miserable, and you'll be setting yourself up for all the
diseases that have been linked with America's epidemic
of overweight and obesity—heart disease, stroke, high
blood pressure, and diabetes, to name a depressing few.

At the same time, if you're like me, you're dreading
going through the drill of carefully portioning out your
peanut butter: getting out a measuring spoon, filling it up,
leveling it off, and carefully scooping it out, then repeat-
ing the entire process again. And you'd need to do that
twice a day, every day, for as long as you follow the
Peanut Butter Diet.

Even I think that's very boring. And very time-consuming.

A PING-PONG BALL TO THE RESCUE

That's why I'm so thrilled to have found an alternative for measuring peanut butter. All you need to do is get a Ping-Pong ball and keep it on your kitchen counter. Then, whenever you want 2 tablespoons of peanut butter, use a regular kitchen spoon to dig a glob of peanut butter about the same size as your Ping-Pong ball out of the jar. It works perfectly, because as I've learned, the volume of a Ping-Pong ball is almost exactly the same as the volume of 2 measuring tablespoons.

Want proof? Let's do the math. The volume of 2 measuring tablespoons is 29.6 cubic centimeters. The official size of a Ping-Pong ball is 3.8 centimeters in diameter, or 1.9 centimeters in radius. Plug that dimension into the formula for the volume of a sphere (if you're among the mathematically inclined, it's volume equals pi—or 3.14— times the radius cubed), and you'll see that the volume of a Ping-Pong ball is 28.7 cubic centimeters. In other words, there's next to no difference in size between a Ping-Pong ball, at 28.7 cubic centimeters, and 2 tablespoons of peanut butter, at 29.6 cubic centimeters!

> **DID YOU KNOW . . .**
>
> The average child will eat 1,500 peanut butter and jelly sandwiches by the time he graduates from high school.
>
> SOURCE: THE NATIONAL PEANUT BOARD

You can buy Ping-Pong balls at sporting goods stores and retailers like Wal-Mart (where we found a pack of 6 for $1.28). You can find white ones, bright orange ones, and multicolored ones; some even have markings like little baseballs, basketballs, and soccer balls.

Once you purchase your Ping-Pong ball, it's important to use a measuring tablespoon to portion out 2 tablespoons of peanut butter at least once. This will convince you that 2 tablespoons really is the equivalent of a Ping-Pong ball. It will also help you learn to eyeball the right serving size when you start using a regular spoon to dig out your peanut butter.

And I do urge you to keep that Ping-Pong ball on the counter, where you can see it. It will keep you honest. I glance at mine to compare it with every spoonful of peanut butter I take.

TABLE TENNIS TRIVIA

Sooner or later, somebody is bound to ask you why you have a Ping-Pong ball sitting on your kitchen counter. After explaining how the ball helps you stick with the Peanut Butter Diet, you can further dazzle your guest with these fascinating facts.

- Invented in England in the early 20th century, table tennis was originally called Ping-Pong, which to this day is protected by trademark. The name *table tennis* was adopted in 1921.
- While we Americans play table tennis as a recreational sport, in Europe and Asia, it's highly organized and competitive.
- Table tennis became an Olympic sport in 1988.

WILL A GOLF BALL DO?

Chances are, you're more likely to have a golf ball around the house than a Ping-Pong ball. And you just might be thinking, "They sure seem like the same size to me!" They are close, but a golf ball is actually one-third larger, at 40.6 cubic centimeters.

Up until now, the golf ball has more or less been the standard model for teaching consumers just how large a 2-tablespoon serving is. Even *Prevention* magazine, where I'm the nutrition editor, has used it. But since we're dealing with something as highly caloric as peanut butter, I've decided that we should rely on a Ping-Pong ball, which is more accurate for portion control.

If you opt for golf ball-size portions, keep in mind that you'll be getting at least 60 extra calories per serving. To keep that from happening, please make sure that your peanut butter glob is the size of a golf ball on a diet!

CALORIE CONTROL GUARANTEED

As long as you use the Ping-Pong ball as your guide to the proper serving size, you'll be able to enjoy the delicious Peanut Butter Diet—rich in healthy and satisfying monounsaturated fat—and still control calories enough to lose weight. My colleagues and I have already done all the tricky calorie counting for you. So you can just dig in and enjoy!

Now that you know how much peanut butter to eat, you may be wondering which kind of peanut butter to eat. Is natural peanut butter better for you than the emulsified varieties sold in supermarkets? In the next chapter, I'll give you the surprising answers.

CHAPTER NINE

Does Brand Matter?

Since the Peanut Butter Diet has so many potential health benefits, you'd naturally want to buy the peanut butter that's the healthiest, too. You certainly have enough brands and kinds to choose from. But which one is best may surprise you.

Perhaps you prefer the "natural" or "old-fashioned" varieties, made from peanut butter and sometimes salt—and that's it. From experience, I know that stirring the oil on the top into the solids on the bottom is a pretty sloppy job. I always get oil spilling down the outside of the jar. And I often wind up with a spread that tends to be either oily or dry, instead of right between.

Then again, maybe you avoid the mess of mixing by sticking with the emulsified brands, such as Skippy, Jif, and Peter Pan. These are already mixed, and they stay that way in the jar. But these brands are rumored to pack lots of added sugar, not to mention unhealthy trans fats.

So which should you choose? Actually, I used to be right on the fence. I'd buy natural until I got tired of mixing it. Then I'd buy emulsified until I got too worried about the trans fats.

Trans fats are present in any food that has partially hydrogenated vegetable oil in its ingredients list. In emulsified peanut butters, the addition of partially hydrogenated oil, such as soybean oil, keeps the peanut solids and peanut oil permanently mixed, so you don't have to do it yourself.

The concern is this: Studies now prove that when ⸱ sumed in high quantities, trans fats are as unhealthy cholesterol readings as saturated fat, and possibly n so. Diets high in trans fats elevate bad LDL cholest⸱ just as saturated fat does. But they also lower good H cholesterol, something saturated fat does not do. heart-healthy diet, we'd be smart to limit consumptio foods high in trans fats.

TESTING FOR TRANS FATS

Like a lot of people, I believed that emulsified peanut ters pack a hefty amount of trans fats. You can ima, my interest when, back in 1999, I received the results study conducted by The Peanut Institute, a peanut in⸱ try trade group. The institute had sent several nati⸱ brands and store brands of emulsified peanut butter t⸱ independent nutrient analysis laboratory to be tested their trans fat content.

To my pleasant surprise, the results showed that e⸱ brand analyzed had ultra-low levels of trans fats. In ⸱

QUICK TIP
To make mixing natural peanut butter a little less messy, try using chopsticks.

they were at least 100 ti⸱ lower than 0.5 gram per ⸱ blespoons, the level at wh⸱ under a proposed FDA ⸱ beling law, a manufact⸱

could describe a product as trans fat–free.

It seemed too good to be true. So just to make s⸱ my *Prevention* magazine colleagues and I sent our ⸱ samples of popular national and store brands to a dif⸱ ent independent testing laboratory. Guess what? Our ⸱ sults were identical to those obtained by The Pe⸱ Institute: All of the brands had trans fats levels at l⸱

100 times lower than what the FDA has defined as trans fat-free.

True, emulsified peanut butters do contain some trans fats. You can see the partially hydrogenated oil right on the ingredients lists. Natural peanut butters, on the other hand, contain no trans fats because they're not made with partially hydrogenated oil.

But as we now know, the trans fat content of emulsified peanut butters is so low that it's insignificant. Many foods fare much worse, especially some packaged foods like cookies, crackers, and snack cakes, as well as frozen entrées, stick margarines, and fast-food french fries.

STAY OUT OF THE REDUCED-FAT TRAP

If you've shopped your supermarket's peanut butter section lately, you've probably noticed that many brands are available in reduced-fat varieties. You may even be using one yourself.

Personally, I don't recommend them. Compared with regular peanut butter, they do have less fat per serving, but that means you're getting less of the heart-healthy monounsaturated fat that helps make peanut butter so good for you.

And here's the real kicker: To replace the fat they remove, manufacturers add forms of sugar, such as corn syrup solids. These sugars bump up the number of calories per serving, so you're getting just about as many as you would if you ate regular peanut butter.

The bottom line: Going with the reduced-fat varieties really doesn't gain you much.

A SWEET SURPRISE ABOUT SUGAR

Even if the trans fats in emulsified peanut butters are no big deal, what about all the added sugars? Indeed, if you look at the ingredients lists of various brands, you'll see sugar and sometimes even molasses (natural peanut butters contain neither). No one wants tons of empty calories from added sugars, especially not people who are trying to lose weight.

But as with trans fats, the big question is: Just how *much* sugar do emulsified peanut butters contain? To get an answer, no laboratory tests are required. The information is right there in plain sight, on the Nutrition Facts panel of every jar of peanut butter in the supermarket. Manufacturers are required to list the grams of sugar per serving.

> **DID YOU KNOW . . .**
>
> Two peanut farmers have been elected president of the United States: Thomas Jefferson and Jimmy Carter.
>
> SOURCE: THE NATIONAL PEANUT BOARD

If you look at the label on a jar of natural peanut butter, you'll see that it has some sugar. But it's not the kind that's added in manufacturing; rather, it's the kind that occurs naturally in peanuts. It amounts to just 2 grams per 2-tablespoon serving. That's about ⅖ teaspoon—so that's wonderful.

You might expect emulsified peanut butters, the ones with added sugars, to fare much worse. Yet labels show that most of them contain only 3 grams of sugar per 2-tablespoon serving. That's about ⅗ teaspoon.

In other words, emulsified peanut butters, which are supposed to be so loaded with added sugars, have only ⅕ teaspoon more sugar per serving than natural peanut butters. That ⅕ teaspoon equals about 3 extra calories, a negligible difference.

SUIT YOURSELF

So the question remains: Which should you choose, natural peanut butter or emulsified peanut butter? That's really up to you. As we've seen, both kinds are equally healthy. The decision just may come down to taste and convenience.

For myself, I haven't bought a jar of natural peanut butter since I learned that the sugar and trans fats in emulsified peanut butter are so negligible. I like the convenience and texture of the good old emulsified brands. My neighbor, on the other hand, would never part with her natural brand. To each her own!

THE TASTERS' CHOICE

When *Cook's Illustrated* magazine asked 20 staff members to taste-test three natural and five emulsified peanut butters, the emulsified brands stole the show. They were rated best in taste right from the jar, best in taste used in peanut sauces, and best in taste used in cookies. In assessing the peanut sauces, the testers observed that the natural peanut butters imparted a grainy texture instead of the silky texture typical of the emulsified peanut butters.

CHAPTER TEN

A 4-Week Plan for
Peanut Butter Indulgence

You're about to embark on an eating plan that will help you lose weight while satisfying your hunger with one of America's richest yet most nutritious comfort foods.

While you're watching the pounds melt away, you'll be keeping your heart healthy, possibly even more so than if you were following a low-fat diet. You'll protect yourself against high blood pressure and diabetes—or, if you already have either condition, you'll be able to manage it better. And you just may reduce your risk of cancer.

Besides two servings a day of peanut butter, you'll be getting nine servings a day of fruits and vegetables, plus whole grains, beans, fish, and calcium-rich foods.

That's one fabulous eating plan. And it's one you can stick with because it's so . . . well, peanut buttery. Remember, women get 4 tablespoons of peanut butter a day, and men get 6.

While almost anyone can try the Peanut Butter Diet, research suggests that it can be especially beneficial for those who weigh more than they should or who have high cholesterol or high triglycerides, high blood pressure, diabetes or insulin resistance, or Syndrome X. Even if you don't need to slim down but have been avoiding peanut butter for fear that it would pack on the pounds, these calorie-controlled eating plans can let you relax and enjoy it again.

Before you start the Peanut Butter Diet, however, please be sure you've read chapter 3. It identifies circumstances in which the diet should be used with caution, if not avoided altogether. While the Peanut Butter Diet can help many people, it's not appropriate for everyone.

WATCH THE WEIGHT DISAPPEAR

If slimming down is your goal, the Peanut Butter Diet can do an amazing job of taking off unwanted pounds—but not because peanut butter contains some miracle compound or secret ingredient. Granted, it may make you feel full longer. But the Peanut Butter Diet works primarily because it controls your calorie intake. "To lose weight, you must cut calories," affirms Jim Glaser, R.D., a nutritionist for Canyon Ranch Health Resort in Tucson. "You can't rely on 'magic' foods or food combinations."

What's more, for weight loss to last, you need to take off the pounds gradually. We at *Prevention* magazine recommend a rate of ½ pound a week, which adds up to 25 pounds a year. For the average woman who's overweight, that means limiting calorie intake to about 1,500 calories a day; the average man who's overweight can go a little higher, to about 2,200 calories a day.

My colleagues and I are convinced that plans promising more rapid weight loss, in the range of 1 to 2 pounds a week—which is most diets—can actually sabotage your efforts. They do this in two ways.

They leave you feeling deprived. To shed pounds that rapidly, you'd have to cut your calorie intake much further than the Peanut Butter Diet recommends—if you're a woman, to around 1,200 calories or less, for example. Sure, you can live that way for a while. But if you're like most people, you'll eventually start feeling deprived. It's as if you're being set up to overeat. And when you do, back come the pounds. By slimming down more gradually, you won't be battling deprivation, which means you're more likely to stick with it.

They rob you of muscle. According to my colleague Michele Stanten, *Prevention*'s fitness editor, when you go the slow-and-steady route to weight loss, you shed mostly excess fat. More rapid weight loss takes away muscle mass as well. As you'll learn in chapter 15, your body needs up to 15 times more calories to support muscle tissue than fat tissue. So you want to hold on to all the muscle you can!

THE DETAILS OF THE DIET

In part 4 of this book, you'll find two sets of detailed 4-week menu plans. The plans in chapter 11 are designed for women and provide 1,500 calories a day; the men's versions in chapter 12 allow for 2,200 calories a day.

Practically speaking, the two sets of plans are almost identical. Sometimes the guys get double and triple servings of foods; occasionally their plans include foods that don't appear in the women's versions at all.

But in both the 1,500- and 2,200-calorie levels, the proportion of total fat, monounsaturated fat, saturated fat, carbohydrates, and protein is the same as that used in studies supporting the health benefits of high-monounsaturated-fat diets. And because the men's and women's plans for any given day are so similar, couples should have no trouble preparing and following the Peanut Butter Diet together.

In designing the menus, the top concern for my colleagues and me—after healthfulness and taste—was convenience. That's why every meal and snack is so super-easy.

Each day's plan features two dishes that use peanut butter, with page numbers that refer you to the corresponding recipes in chapter 13.

In many cases, the "recipes" are completely fuss-free favorites like peanut butter melted on a toasted English muffin or spread on apple slices. You'll even notice some childhood treats like S'Mores.

Occasionally, you will come across recipes with longer lists of ingredients. Don't panic. All of the dishes are quick to prepare; I insisted on it. Part of the charm of peanut butter is its utter convenience. Why spoil things with time-consuming meal preparation? That's why, whenever we could, we took advantage of other healthy "convenience foods" as well, such as precooked chicken breast meat and frozen whole-grain waffles.

We also designed many of the recipes to make just one or two servings. That way, you won't end up with a family's worth of food if it's just you and your significant other (or you and your dog or cat).

Please note that not all of the recipes in chapter 13 appear in the menu plans. Sometimes we discovered a quick-and-healthy peanut butter dish so delicious that we couldn't resist passing it along to you. Some of the recipes are ideal when company's coming; I'll point those out as well.

> **DID YOU KNOW . . .**
>
> Adults actually eat more peanut butter than children do.
>
> SOURCE: THE NATIONAL PEANUT BOARD

In any given menu plan, if you want to swap one peanut butter recipe for another, that's okay. Just be sure the replacement has, at most, 25 calories more than the original. You'll find that information in the nutrient analysis provided with every recipe.

THE FIRST STEPS TO WEIGHT-LOSS SUCCESS

I know that all of this may seem a bit overwhelming at the moment. But once you get into the menu plans and recipes, you'll realize just how easy the Peanut Butter Diet is. You'll love it even more—and give yourself the best chance for weight-loss success—if you start out on the right foot. Just follow these simple steps.

I. Decide how much you need to lose. To determine a realistic goal for yourself, check out "What's Your BMI?" on page 97. "BMI" stands for body mass index, which many experts feel is the most accurate gauge of ideal weight—much better than the bathroom scale.

If you need to drop more than 20 pounds, I recommend setting an interim goal of 10 pounds and, when you achieve it, maintaining that loss for a while. Once you feel comfortable there, you can try for another 10 pounds. Continue in 10-pound increments until you reach your ideal weight.

Throughout this process, keep in mind that a loss of just 10 pounds helps reduce your risk for heart disease, high blood pressure, and diabetes.

2. Take the Ping-Pong Pledge. I can't say it enough: Portion control is absolutely essential to the success of the Peanut Butter Diet. As you'll recall from chapter 8, I recommend gauging your peanut butter portions with help from a Ping-Pong ball. Don't even start the diet until you have that ball sitting on your kitchen counter.

3. Choose the right calorie level. If you're a woman, you'll want to use the 1,500-calorie menu plans presented

in chapter 11. If you're a man, turn to the plans in chapter 12, each of which provides 2,200 calories.

4. Read the recipe directions carefully. Each menu plan includes page numbers that direct you to the recipes for particular peanut butter dishes. Just keep in mind that a recipe may have two sets of directions. The basic recipe is for women; men need to adjust the amounts of some of the ingredients as noted. If you see two asterisks (**), that means men should double the amount; three asterisks (***) means triple the amount.

5. Design a different diet. If you get tired of eating peanut butter every day—and most people will, even the peanut butter fanatics—you can still reap the rewards of a satisfying but calorie-controlled high-monounsaturated-fat diet by turning to chapter 14. There you'll find a formula for designing your own menus using other sources of monounsaturated fat, such as olive oil, avocados, and other nuts. You'll also get two sample menus to start you off.

Even though the Peanut Butter Diet includes a healthy mix of foods, you'll get even greater variety by trying different foods rich in monounsaturated fat. Variety makes dietitians very happy.

6. Come back for a peanut butter fix. Whether for a day, a week, or a month, you can resume the Peanut Butter Diet whenever you wish. The menu plans and recipes will be waiting for you, so you can indulge in peanut butter without fear of putting on pounds.

7. If you need to, *stop*. If you try the Peanut Butter Diet for 2 weeks and find that you're consistently eating more peanut butter than you should, this is not the right diet for you. For some people, peanut butter is a trigger food that

WHAT'S YOUR BMI?

To determine whether you should lose weight, and how much, you should figure out your body mass index, or BMI. It involves using a simple formula that takes into consideration both your current weight and your height. Just get out your calculator and do the math.

1. Multiply your weight in pounds (measured while you're wearing underwear but no shoes) by 703.
2. Divide the total by your height (in inches).
3. Divide that figure by your height (in inches).

The number you get is your BMI.

As an example, let's say you are 5 feet 7 inches tall (67 inches) and you weigh 170 pounds. Plug those numbers into the BMI formula.

$$170 \times 703 = 119,510$$
$$119,510 \div 67 = 1,784$$
$$1,784 \div 67 = 26.6$$

In this example, your BMI is 26.6.

Now calculate your actual BMI using your real height and weight. To find out if it's considered "healthy," "overweight," or "obese," just locate your number in the following BMI chart. (You can also find your BMI in the chart if you'd rather not do the math yourself. Just look at the top of the column where your height and weight intersect.)

If your BMI is within the healthy range, good for you! The Peanut Butter Diet can help you stay there.

If your BMI is in the overweight or obese range, you're at greater risk for serious health problems such as heart disease, stroke, diabetes, and some cancers. I urge you to do what you can to get your BMI lower. The Peanut Butter Diet can help you achieve that goal.

they just can't help overeating, even when they have it every day. Don't think of it as failing. You've just learned a valuable lesson: In order to reach a healthy weight, you should probably keep peanut butter out of your home.

BODY MASS INDEX						
			HEALTHY			
BMI	19	20	21	22	23	24
HEIGHT (in)			WEIGHT (lb)			
58	91	96	100	105	110	115
59	94	99	104	109	114	119
60	97	102	107	112	118	123
61	100	106	111	116	122	127
62	104	109	115	120	125	131
63	107	113	118	124	130	135
64	110	116	122	128	134	140
65	114	120	126	132	138	144
66	118	124	130	136	142	148
67	121	127	134	140	146	153
68	125	131	138	144	151	158
69	128	135	142	149	155	162
70	132	139	146	153	160	167
71	136	143	150	157	165	172
72	140	147	154	162	169	177
73	144	151	159	166	174	182
74	148	155	163	171	179	186
75	152	160	168	176	184	192
76	156	164	172	180	189	197

WHAT TO DO WHEN THE POUNDS WON'T GO

Let's suppose you've been following the Peanut Butter Diet religiously but you've not lost as much as you've expected. Ask yourself these questions.

Are you eating tennis balls instead of Ping-Pong balls of peanut butter? Try portioning out exactly 2 measuring tablespoons' worth of peanut butter. If you've been eating more than that, you've been getting extra calories. Be

BODY MASS INDEX (cont'd)

OVERWEIGHT					OBESE		
25	26	27	28	29	30	31	32
WEIGHT (lb)					WEIGHT (lb)		
119	124	129	134	138	143	148	153
124	128	133	138	143	148	153	158
128	133	138	143	148	153	158	163
132	137	143	148	153	158	164	169
136	142	147	153	158	164	169	175
141	146	152	158	163	169	175	180
145	151	157	163	169	174	180	186
150	156	162	168	174	180	186	192
155	161	167	173	179	186	192	198
159	166	172	178	185	191	198	204
164	171	177	184	190	197	203	210
169	176	182	189	196	203	209	216
174	181	188	195	202	209	216	222
179	186	193	200	208	215	222	229
184	191	199	206	213	221	228	235
189	197	204	212	219	227	235	242
194	202	210	218	225	233	241	249
200	208	216	224	232	240	248	256
205	213	221	230	238	246	254	263

SOURCE: National Institutes of Health

honest with yourself. Underestimating portion sizes of high-calorie foods is very common—and very human.

Are you getting enough vitamin X? That's X as in "x-ercise." You know, physical activity. Moving around. The calorie levels of the Peanut Butter Diet assume that you are engaging in at least 30 minutes of activity

DID YOU KNOW . . .

When making a PB&J sandwich, 96 percent of people put on the peanut butter before the jelly.

SOURCE: THE NATIONAL PEANUT BOARD

three times a week and that it's vigorous enough to raise your heart rate. In fact, the federal government's updated dietary guidelines for weight loss or maintenance recommend 45 minutes of physical activity 7 days a week. So do we at *Prevention* magazine. In chapter 15, I'll talk more about easy ways to incorporate exercise into your day.

In the meantime, start thinking of any opportunity to move your body as a luxury that is threatened by modern technology. See yourself as "movement-deprived." Look at even routine activities like making the bed or taking out the trash as priceless, vanishing commodities—because they are. All of us must get moving.

Are you a woman who's under 5 feet 2? Women who are very petite may need to cut their calorie consumption even more in order to lose weight. If this describes you, be sure to read chapter 14. It will show you how you can modify the Peanut Butter Diet to provide just 1,200 calories a day instead of 1,500. This low calorie intake is not recommended for people who are taller, however.

PART IV

Dig In to the Diet

CHAPTER ELEVEN

The Menu Plans for Women

Get set to dig in to 4 weeks of fabulously healthy, peanut buttery menu plans that provide about 1,500 calories a day. For the average woman, following these menu plans should produce weight loss of about ½ pound a week, or 25 pounds over the course of a year. If slimming down is your goal, don't forget that you also need your vitamin X—45 minutes of accumulated physical activity every day. (It's easier than you think, as you'll see in chapter 15.)

Each day's menu includes two generous 2-tablespoon servings of peanut butter, or 4 tablespoons total. They're incorporated into fuss-free but utterly delicious recipes like Peanut Butter Hot Chocolate or Peanut Butter Oatmeal. The page number for each super-easy recipe is given right in the menu. And once you learn to use a Ping-Pong ball as your portion-control model, you can measure out 2 tablespoons of peanut butter in a snap.

MAKING CHANGES

If and when you want a change from eating peanut butter every day, just turn to chapter 14. There you'll learn an easy formula for designing delectable 1,500-calorie menus using other sources of healthy monounsaturated fats, including olive oil, canola oil, peanuts and other nuts, and avocados. You'll find sample menus for those diets, too.

Whenever you need a peanut butter fix, though, you'll

always have these healthy, calorie-controlled menu plans to come back to. You can satisfy your peanut butter cravings for a day, a week, or a month, without sacrificing your trim body or your health.

If you find that some days' menu plans fit your lifestyle better than others, feel free to repeat them more frequently. But remember that for maximum health, the more variety your diet has, the better off you are.

You may also find that you prefer certain peanut butter treats and recipes over others. In that case, you can substitute one peanut butter dish for another as long as the

---

SUPPLEMENTS FOR INSURANCE

The Peanut Butter Diet delivers a wealth of nutrients, including some that people tend to run low on. For extra nutritional support, you may want to consider taking the following:

A daily multivitamin: *Prevention* magazine advises every adult to take a daily multivitamin/mineral supplement, one that supplies approximately 100 percent of the Daily Values for most vitamins and minerals. Even though the Peanut Butter Diet menu plans are ultrahealthy, I think it makes sense to have a multi make up for any potential nutritional shortfalls.

Calcium: Many of the menu plans provide approximately 1,000 milligrams of calcium a day, the recommended amount for people under age 50. If you are 50 or older, you should be getting 1,200 milligrams a day, and some experts recommend 1,500 milligrams. In this case, you'll need a separate calcium supplement that supplies 200 to 500 milligrams a day. Most multivitamins do not contain this much.

Vitamin D: If you are age 70 or older, you need extra vitamin D. Most multivitamins provide 400 international units. Once you're in your seventies, your recommended daily intake increases to 600 IU. Try to find a calcium supplement that contains an additional 200 IU of vitamin D.

replacement doesn't exceed the original by more than about 25 calories.

THE SUPER STATS

In the Peanut Butter Diet, each day's menu includes an incredibly nutritious nine servings of vegetables and fruits. Scientists are identifying more and more natural compounds in veggies and fruits that seem to have the power to help fight cancer, heart disease, cataracts, and a host of other health concerns. In fact, some experts theorize that eventually we'll view illnesses like cancer as "deficiency diseases" caused by not eating enough nutritious plant foods.

You've probably heard that you should aim for at least 5 servings of fruits and vegetables a day, but cutting-edge research suggests that a higher intake is really optimal. The famous DASH (Dietary Approaches to Stop Hypertension) diet to lower blood pressure, now recommended by the National Institutes of Health, provides for 8 to 10 servings of fruits and vegetables a day. Preliminary studies involving women at high risk for breast cancer found that after just 2 weeks of eating 8 or more servings of veggies and fruits every day, the amount of DNA damage in the women's cells—thought to be a marker for cancer risk—had dropped dramatically.

Here's another super stat: On the Peanut Butter Diet, women get about 29 grams of fiber a day. That's more than double the average intake. High-fiber diets seem to help reduce the risk of heart attack, stroke, and cancer. Plus, fiber may be a calorie-eater: In one study, every extra gram of fiber people ate stopped their bodies from absorbing about 7 calories.

Although none of our Peanut Butter Diet menus have identical nutritional profiles, they average out as follows.

- 35 percent of calories from fat—16 percent monounsaturated fat, 13 percent polyunsaturated fat, and 7 percent saturated fat
- 50 percent of calories from carbohydrates (vegetables, fruits, beans, and grains)
- 15 percent of calories from protein, including the cholesterol-free protein in peanut butter

That's very close to the ratio of fat, monounsaturated fat, carbohydrates, and protein used in studies like the one at Pennsylvania State University, which show that a calorie-controlled diet higher in monounsaturated fat

---

A WORD ABOUT SALT

These days, one of the most controversial subjects among health experts is salt intake. Many authorities, including the National Institutes of Health and the American Heart Association, recommend consuming no more than 2,400 milligrams of sodium a day. But others believe salt restriction is important only for those who are salt-sensitive—that is, whose blood pressure rises when they eat a high-salt diet. Some experts also point to evidence that eating a diet with adequate potassium and magnesium, such as the Peanut Butter Diet, helps lower high blood pressure more effectively than restricting salt.

So how much salt will you get when you follow the Peanut Butter Diet? The women's menus average about 2,400 milligrams daily. But because we've tried to use convenience foods to make the diet practical and easy, the men's menus average about 3,000 milligrams a day. By choosing a no-salt-added peanut butter, you can reduce this amount by at least 400 milligrams a day.

But if your doctor has advised you to restrict your sodium intake to 2,400 milligrams or less a day, for any reason, you should discuss the Peanut Butter Diet with him before you try it.

may actually be better for your heart than a low-fat diet. So sticking with the Peanut Butter Diet just may do your health—and your waistline—a world of good!

DAY 1: MONDAY

Breakfast
Peanut Butter Oatmeal (page 192)

Lunch
Bean burrito, restaurant or homemade (for homemade, combine an 8" tortilla, ½ cup beans, and 3 Tbsp salsa)
   1 cup bell pepper strips, baby carrots, or other vegetable of your choice
   ¾ cup calcium-enriched V-8

Snack
1 cup fruit salad

Dinner
Chicken and vegetable stir-fry (2 cups vegetables, 2 oz chicken—a scant ½ cup). In a Chinese restaurant, ask for very little oil. A safer bet, calorie-wise: Sauté 1 tsp each minced ginger and garlic with 2 cups fresh or frozen veggie mix containing broccoli in 1 tsp canola or peanut oil. Add your own chicken (precooked chicken like Perdue Short Cuts is fine). Season with teriyaki sauce.
   ½ cup cookedbrown rice (instant is fine)

Evening Treat
S'More (page 200)
   1,453 calories, 71 g protein, 188 g carbohydrates, 53 g fat, 12 g saturated fat, 24 g monounsaturated fat, 29 g fiber, 2,486 mg sodium, 832 mg calcium

DAY 2: TUESDAY

Breakfast
1 oz whole grain or bran cereal—should be 110 to 130 calories per ¾ to 1 cup, with at least 5 g fiber (Kellogg's Complete Wheat Bran Flakes and Kashi Good Friends are good choices)—with 1 small banana, sliced, and 1 cup fat-free milk (if this is too much milk for your bowl, drink the rest separately)

   ¾ cup calcium-fortified citrus juice

Lunch
Peanut Butter, Ham, and Pickle Sandwich (page 195)

   1 cup cherry tomatoes and celery sticks
   ¾ cup calcium-enriched V-8

Snack
½ cup red pepper slices dipped in ¼ cup bean dip (canned, or mash a heaping ¼ cup canned black beans with a dash of cumin, black pepper, and a few drops of olive oil) and 2 to 4 Tbsp salsa. Optional: chopped cilantro

Dinner
4 oz broiled fish of your choice

   1 cup (about 8 spears) steamed asparagus with a dash of lemon juice

   ½ cup whole wheat couscous combined with 2 Tbsp raisins

Evening Treat
Peanut Butter Pudding in a Flash (page 180)

   1,492 calories, 84 g protein, 212 g carbohydrates, 42 g

fat, 9 g saturated fat, 18 g monounsaturated fat, 34 g fiber, 4,546 sodium, 826 mg calcium

DAY 3: WEDNESDAY

Breakfast
Mushroom scrambled eggs: In a nonstick pan, sauté ½ cup chopped mushrooms and 1 chopped scallion (optional) in 1 tsp olive or canola oil until wilted. Add 2 eggs and salt and pepper to taste. Serve on a toasted whole wheat or oat bran English muffin.
   ¾ cup calcium-enriched citrus juice

Lunch
Grilled chicken salad: In a restaurant, ask for dressing on the side and use the dip/spear method—dip your fork in the dressing, then spear a bite of salad. A safer bet, calorie-wise: Toss 3 cups greens with 1 Tbsp reduced-fat olive- or canola-oil-based dressing of your choice (Annie's Naturals Low-Fat Gingerly Vinaigrette is a good one), then add 3 oz grilled, skinless chicken strips (Perdue Short Cuts are fine).

Snack
Peanut Butter–Stuffed Celery (page 183)

Dinner
1 cup whole wheat spaghetti with ⅓ cup marinara sauce and 1 Tbsp Parmesan cheese
   2 cups microwaved cauliflower, tossed with a dash of lemon, 1 tsp olive oil, and 1 Tbsp Parmesan

Evening Treat
Peanut Butter Hot Chocolate (page 196)

1,484 calories, 96 g protein, 145 g carbohydrates, 66 g fat, 15 g saturated fat, 29 g monounsaturated fat, 25 g fiber, 1,856 mg sodium, 1,078 mg calcium

DAY 4: THURSDAY

Breakfast
Peanut Butter Breakfast Shake (page 194)

½ cup diced cantaloupe

Lunch
Turkey sandwich: 2 oz sliced turkey breast with mustard, lettuce, and tomato on whole grain bread

Salad: 2 cups greens, 1 cup other vegetables, 1 Tbsp reduced-fat olive- or canola-oil-based dressing

Snack
1 cup plain fat-free yogurt with ½ tsp maple syrup and a dash of vanilla extract

Dinner
⅔ cup Peanut Butter Creole Soup (page 197)

1 cup Cajun beans and rice: Use any mix, such as Uncle Ben's Chef's Recipe, with about 210 calories per cup. Add 1 cup mixed vegetables (such as frozen peas and carrots, thawed).

½ cup cucumber slices with salt to taste

Evening Treat
2 dates, chopped and mixed in 4-oz container of fat-free tapioca pudding

1,489 calories, 85 g protein, 215 g carbohydrates, 40 g fat, 9 g saturated fat, 17 g monounsaturated fat, 29 g fiber, 1,950 mg sodium, 1,272 mg calcium

DAY 5: FRIDAY

Breakfast
Peanut Butter–Frosted Energy Bar (page 194)
   1 cup fat-free milk, plain or in café latte
   2 tangerines or 1 large wedge of cantaloupe

Lunch
⅔ cup Peanut Butter Creole Soup (page 197, or microwave last night's leftovers)
   Salad bar: At least 2 cups raw greens, 1½ cups other raw vegetables, 1 hard-boiled egg (or 3 Tbsp chopped egg), and ½ cup beans (such as chickpeas or kidney beans), tossed with 2 Tbsp reduced-calorie olive- or canola-oil-based dressing
   1 slice whole wheat bread

Snack
Orange "soda": ¾ cup calcium-fortified citrus juice mixed with ½ cup seltzer

Dinner
2 slices pizza—ask for light cheese and lots of extra veggies (each slice: ⅛ of 12" pizza, about 140 calories per slice, including ½ cup veggies per slice)
   ½ cup cucumber slices with salt to taste
   8 oz light beer

Evening Treat
½ cup strawberries
   1,536 calories, 67 g protein, 204 g carbohydrates, 52 g

fat, 12 g saturated fat, 22 g monounsaturated fat, 29 g fiber, 1,630 mg sodium, 1,220 mg calcium

DAY 6: SATURDAY

Breakfast
Peanut Butter Maple Syrup Waffles (page 202)
   1 cup fat-free milk, plain or in café latte

Lunch
Tuna salad: Combine half of a 6-oz can drained, water-packed, white albacore tuna with 2 tsp reduced-calorie mayonnaise, ½ tsp Dijon mustard, and 2 Tbsp finely chopped carrots and celery. Optional: 1 tsp chopped pickles.
   1½ cups baby carrots, red bell pepper strips
   ¾ cup calcium-enriched V-8

Snack
Orange, pear, or other fruit of your choice

Dinner
Tahitian Chicken with Peanut Butter Mango Sauce (page 175), served over ½ cup cooked rice (preferably brown basmati)
   ½ cup cooked spinach

Evening Treat
1½"-thick slice angel food cake topped with 1½ cups coarsely mashed strawberries
   1,504 calories, 89 g protein, 183 g carbohydrates, 52 g fat, 11 g saturated fat, 23 g monounsaturated fat, 26 g fiber, 2,091 mg sodium, 1,059 mg calcium

DAY 7: SUNDAY

Breakfast
Peanut Butter French Toast (page 200)
   ¾ cup calcium-enriched citrus juice

Lunch
Mediterranean salad: Combine ½ cup each chickpeas, chopped tomatoes, cucumbers, and red or green bell peppers. Mix with 2 Tbsp fresh basil (or 1 tsp dried), 2 tsp olive oil, and a scant tsp lemon juice. Add salt and pepper to taste.
   1 slice crusty whole grain bread, brushed with ¼ tsp olive oil and grilled or toasted

Snack
6 baked tortilla chips dipped in 2 to 4 Tbsp salsa

Dinner
Chicken Kebabs with Chinese Peanut Butter Sauce (page 170)
   ½ cup cooked brown rice (instant is fine)
   Yogurt cucumber salad: Combine ¾ cup plain fat-free yogurt with ¼ cup finely chopped cucumbers, ½ tsp dried mint, and a dash of garlic powder or ¼ tsp fresh garlic.

Evening Treat
1 cup strawberries
   1,525 calories, 81 g protein, 199 g carbohydrates, 51 g fat, 12 g saturated fat, 22 g monounsaturated fat, 27 g fiber, 1,758 g sodium, 882 mg calcium

DAY 8: MONDAY

Breakfast
1 oz whole grain or bran cereal—should be 110 to 130 calories per ¾ to 1 cup, with at least 5 g fiber (Kashi Go Lean and Barbara's Puffins are good choices)—with 1 small banana, sliced, and 1 cup fat-free milk (if this is too much milk for your bowl, drink the rest separately)

Lunch
Turkey-avocado bagel: Fill a 3- to 4-oz whole wheat or oat bran bagel with 2 oz sliced turkey, ¼ avocado, sliced, lettuce, and tomato slices.
   ¾ cup calcium-enriched V-8
   1 cup fruit salad

Snack
1 small cookie (2½" diameter) of your choice with tea, herbal tea, or coffee

Dinner
Cold Peanut Butter Noodles (page 182)
   Spinach and carrot salad: Toss together 3 cups spinach leaves, 1 carrot, grated, and 1 chopped scallion. Combine ½ tsp low-sodium soy sauce, ½ tsp honey, 1 tsp canola oil (for a blander flavor) or olive oil (for a stronger flavor), and ½ tsp lemon juice. Toss with the salad.

Evening Treat
Peanut Butter–Stuffed Celery (page 183)
   1,471 calories, 70 g protein, 205 g carbohydrates, 52 g fat, 10 g saturated fat, 25 g monounsaturated fat, 28 g fiber, 2,315 mg sodium, 783 mg calcium

DAY 9: TUESDAY

Breakfast
Scrambled egg sandwich: In a nonstick pan, scramble 1 egg and 1 egg white with ½ tsp canola or olive oil. Place between 2 slices whole wheat bread with 3 slices tomato.
   1 cup diced or 1 large wedge cantaloupe
   1 cup fat-free milk, plain or in café latte

Lunch
1 cup lentil, split pea, or black bean soup (canned or instant is fine)
   Salad: 3 cups greens, 1 cup chopped vegetables, with 1½ Tbsp reduced-calorie olive- or canola-oil-based dressing
   ¾ cup calcium-enriched V-8

Snack
Peanut Butter Banana (page 203)

Dinner
Frozen dinner based on chicken—230 to 250 calories, 4 to 6 g fat (examples: Lean Cuisine Café Classics Glazed Chicken or Healthy Choice Grilled Chicken Sonoma)
   1 cup cherry tomatoes

Evening Treat
Angel Food Cake with Peanut Butter "Icing" (page 196)
   1,519 calories, 77 g protein, 203 g carbohydrates, 53 g fat, 11 g saturated fat, 22 g monounsaturated fat, 29 g fiber, 3,124 mg sodium, 668 mg calcium

DAY 10: WEDNESDAY

Breakfast
Peanut Butter Oatmeal (page 192)

Lunch
Salad bar: 3 cups spinach with ½ cup tomato slices; ½ cup cauliflower or other vegetable of your choice; ½ cup chickpeas, kidney beans, or other beans; and 1½ Tbsp reduced-fat olive-oil- or canola-oil-based dressing
   ¾ cup calcium-enriched V-8

Snack
1 small cookie (2½" diameter) of your choice, with tea, herbal tea, or coffee

Dinner
Sweet and Bacon-y Peanut Butter Muffins (page 176)
   Salad: 3 cups Bibb lettuce, ½ cup chopped celery, 1 tangerine, sectoned, 1 chopped scallion, and 1 Tbsp slivered almonds tossed with 1 Tbsp orange juice, 1 tsp olive oil, ½ tsp lemon juice, and salt and pepper to taste

Evening Treat
½ cup frozen yogurt topped with ½ cup coarsely mashed fresh or frozen strawberries
   1,542 calories, 71 g protein, 204 g carbohydrates, 59 g fat, 11 g saturated fat, 28 g monounsaturated fat, 32 g fiber, 2,451 mg sodium, 1,141 mg calcium

DAY 11:THURSDAY

Breakfast
2 mozzarella or string cheese sticks (for example, Polly-O or Sargento, about 70 calories apiece)
  ½ oz whole grain crackers
  1 cup grapes

Lunch
Peanut Butter and Jelly Sandwich (page 168)
  1 cup red pepper slices dipped in ¼ cup plain fat-free yogurt mixed with a dash of garlic salt
  Fruit "soda": ¾ cup fruit juice of your choice combined with ½ cup seltzer

Snack
3 Hershey's Kisses

Dinner
Turkey chili: Sauté ⅓ lb ground turkey with chili seasoning and onions (optional). Combine with 2 cups chopped zucchini, 1 cup canned refried beans, and 1 cup canned or frozen corn. Add water as needed and heat through. (Serves 2; eat just half.)
  ½ cup cooked brown rice (instant is fine)
  ¾ cup calcium-enriched V-8
  Note: Reserve ½ cup corn for tomorrow's lunch.

Evening Treat
Peanut Butter Pudding in a Flash (page 180)
  1,489 calories, 66 g protein, 194 g carbohydrates, 56 g fat, 17 g saturated fat, 23 g monounsaturated fat, 21 g fiber, 1,967 mg sodium, 986 mg calcium

DAY 12: FRIDAY

Breakfast
Peanut Butter Breakfast Shake (page 194)

Lunch
Corn, chicken, and bean salad: Combine ½ cup canned or frozen corn with ½ cup beans of your choice (chickpeas or white cannelloni work well), ½ cup chopped green or red bell peppers, ½ cup chopped or cherry tomatoes, 2 oz chopped chicken (a heaping ⅓ cup; Perdue Short Cuts are a good, quick choice). Toss with 1 Tbsp reduced-fat olive- or canola-oil-based dressing of your choice. Optional: 1 Tbsp fresh cilantro.

1 piece fruit of your choice

Snack
Peanut Butter and Jelly Crackers (page 200)

Dinner
3 to 4 oz broiled or steamed fish of your choice

1½ cups microwaved vegetables tossed with a dash of lemon and salt and pepper to taste

Two ½"-thick slices polenta (buy premade polenta "logs"), each topped with ½ tsp Parmesan cheese and grilled in toaster oven according to polenta package directions (or use 2 large slices crusty whole grain bread)

Evening Treat
Orange Creamsicle: In a blender, whip ¾ cup calcium-enriched orange juice, ¼ cup fat-free milk, ½ tsp vanilla extract, ¼ cup fat-free vanilla frozen yogurt, and 2 ice cubes

1,561 calories, 86 g protein, 205 g carbohydrates, 53 g

fat, 11 g saturated fat, 24 g monounsaturated fat, 28 g fiber, 1,150 mg sodium, 907 mg calcium

DAY 13: SATURDAY

Breakfast
1 egg, fried in 1 tsp olive or canola oil, with 1 slice (1½" thick) cooked polenta
   ¾ cup citrus juice of your choice

Lunch
Peanut Butter Bacon, and Cornbread Squares (page 188)
   1½ cups red bell pepper strips, and celery sticks
   1 cup fat-free milk, plain or in café latte

Snack
1 apple or other fruit of your choice

Dinner
1 cup low-sodium tomato soup simmered with ½ cup peas, chopped carrots, or other vegetable of your choice
   3 oz rotisserie chicken breast (about ½ small breast) from supermarket, skin removed
   Baked potato topped with ½ cup chopped broccoli and ¼ cup plain fat-free yogurt

Evening Treat
Peanut Butter Ice Cream Shake (page 185)
   1,546 calories, 80 g protein, 225 g carbohydrates, 44 g fat, 10 g saturated fat, 18 g monounsaturated fat, 21 g fiber, 1,699 mg sodium, 1,038 mg calcium

DAY 14: SUNDAY

Breakfast

Peanut Butter Cinnamon Toast (page 186)
    1 cup fat-free milk, plain or in café latte
    1 cup sliced strawberries or any other fruit of your choice

Lunch

Tuna salad sandwich on whole wheat. To make tuna
salad: Combine half of a 6-oz can drained, water-packed,
white albacore tuna with 2 tsp reduced-calorie mayonnaise, ½ tsp Dijon mustard, and 2 Tbsp chopped celery.
Optional: 1 tsp chopped pickles.
    1½ cups baby carrots and red bell pepper strips

Snack

¾ cup calcium-enriched V-8

Dinner

Peanut Butter Island Shrimp (page 172)
    ½ cup cooked brown basmati rice (or instant brown rice)
    1 cup microwaved sugar snap peas (frozen are fine)
dressed with ½ tsp olive oil and a dash of lemon juice
    Salad: 2 cups greens, 1 cup cherry tomatoes with 1
Tbsp reduced-fat canola- or olive-oil-based dressing

Evening Treat

2 small cookies (2½" diameter) such as Chips Ahoy soft
cookies (great microwaved) with decaf coffee or tea
    1,482 calories, 90 g protein, 168 g carbohydrates, 57 g
fat, 12 g saturated fat, 25 g monounsaturated fat, 28 g
fiber, 2,972 mg sodium, 935 mg calcium

DAY 15: MONDAY

Breakfast
Peanut Butter–Frosted Energy Bar (page 194)
   1 cup fat-free milk, plain or in café latte
   7 dried apricot halves or 2 Tbsp raisins

Lunch
Peanut Butter and Jelly Sandwich (page 168)
   ½ cup celery sticks

Snack
1 cup fruit salad

Dinner
Bean bruschetta: Heat ¼ cup cannelini beans. Remove from heat and mash coarsely with 1 tsp chopped fresh basil (or ¾ tsp dried) and ¼ tsp olive oil. Grill 1 slice crusty whole grain bread, each brushed with ¼ tsp olive oil. Spread with bean mixture and top with 1 tsp Parmesan cheese.

Greek salad: Toss together ¼ cup white beans, 3 cups greens, 8 cherry tomatoes or 1 medium chopped tomato, ½ cup chopped cucumber, ¼ cup green or red bell pepper slices, and ½ tsp dried oregano. Toss with 2 Tbsp reduced-calorie canola- or olive-oil-based dressing of your choice. Top with 3 Tbsp crumbled feta cheese and 2 olives.

Evening Treat
1 cup fat-free milk, plain or in café latte
   Note: Prepare Gingered Peanut Butter–Carrot Spread (page 185) for next day.

   1,530 calories, 68 g protein, 213 g carbohydrates, 54 g fat, 14 g saturated fat, 22 g monounsaturated fat, 32 g fiber, 1,905 mg sodium, 1,326 mg calcium

DAY 16: TUESDAY

Breakfast
1 oz whole grain or bran cereal—should be 110 to 130 calories per ¾ to 1 cup, with at least 5 g fiber (Kellogg's Complete Wheat Bran Flakes and Kashi Good Friends are good choices)—with 1 small banana, sliced, and 1 cup fat-free milk (if this is too much milk for your bowl, drink the rest separately)

Lunch
Turkey sandwich: 2 oz sliced turkey breast with mustard, lettuce, and tomato on whole grain bread

1 cup red bell pepper strips dipped in Gingered Peanut Butter–Carrot Spread (page 185)

Snack
1 cup fruit salad

Dinner
Veggie burger (Gardenburger, Boca Burger and Amy's California Veggie Burger are all good choices) on whole grain bun with lettuce, 3 slices tomato, ⅛ avocado, and 2 Tbsp crumbled feta cheese

1½ cups microwaved broccoli or other vegetable of your choice, with a dash of lemon

Evening Treat
Peanut Butter Hot Chocolate (page 196)

1,499 calories, 91 g protein, 183 g carbohydrates, 56 g fat, 13 g saturated fat, 23 g monounsaturated fat, 33 g fiber, 2,272 mg sodium, 1,052 mg calcium

DAY 17: WEDNESDAY

Breakfast

Whole wheat or oat bran English muffin, cut in half, toasted, and spread with ½ cup Gingered Peanut Butter–Carrot Spread (page 185)

1 cup fat-free milk, plain or in café latte

1 cup diced or 1 large wedge cantaloupe

Lunch

1 cup lentil, split pea, or black bean soup (canned or instant is fine)

Salad: 3 cups greens, 1 cup chopped vegetables, and 1 Tbsp reduced-fat olive- or canola oil-based dressing

Snack

¾ cup calcium-enriched citrus juice

Dinner

"Kitchen sink" pasta: To 1 cup cooked whole wheat ziti or other short pasta, add 1 cup diced tomatoes, 2 olives, ½ cup cooked, skinless chicken (Perdue Short Cuts are fine), ½ cup microwaved vegetable of your choice (such as broccoli and cauliflower). Toss with 2 tsp olive oil and season with ½ Tbsp chopped fresh basil (or 1 tsp dried). Add salt and pepper to taste.

Evening Treat

Peanut Butter Ice Crean (page 190)

1,516 calories, 78 g protein, 190 g carbohydrates, 58 g fat, 11 g saturated fat, 29 g monounsaturated fat, 29 g fiber, 2,057 mg sodium, 966 mg calcium

DAY 18: THURSDAY

Breakfast
Peanut Butter Bagel (page 000)
    1 cup fruit salad
    1 cup fat-free milk, plain or in café latte

Lunch
Grilled chicken salad: In a restaurant, ask for dressing on the side and use the dip/spear method—dip your fork in the dressing, then spear a bite of salad. A safer bet, calorie-wise: Toss 3 cups greens with 1 Tbsp reduced-fat olive- or canola-oil-based dressing of your choice (Annie's Naturals Low-Fat Gingerly Vinaigrette is a good one), then add 3 oz grilled, skinless chicken strips (Perdue Short Cuts are fine).
    1 orange or other fruit of your choice

Snack
1 small cookie (2½" diameter) of your choice
    1 cup fat-free milk, plain or in café latte

Dinner
Homemade burrito: Heat a 6" to 8" tortilla (preferably whole wheat) and fill with ½ cup canned refried beans, 1 or 2 leaves chopped lettuce, and 2 to 4 Tbsp salsa.
    Mexican grilled vegetables: Skewer 6 regular mushrooms and 1 zucchini (about 5") cut in diagonal slices. Brush with a combo of 2 tsp olive oil, ½ tsp chili powder, 1 tsp lime juice, and ½ clove crushed garlic (optional). Grill (or broil 5" from the broiler) for 5 minutes, turn, brush again, and grill 5 minutes longer, or until softened.

Evening Treat
S'More (page 200)

1,546 calories, 88 g protein, 188 g carbohydrates, 58 g fat, 13 g saturated fat, 27 g monounsaturated fat, 29 g fiber, 2,260 mg sodium, 966 mg calcium

DAY 19: FRIDAY

Breakfast
1 oz whole grain or bran cereal—should be 110 to 130 calories per ¾ to 1 cup, with at least 5 g fiber (Kellogg's Complete Wheat Bran Flakes and Kashi Good Friends are good choices)—with 1 small banana, sliced, and 1 cup fat-free milk (if this is too much milk for your bowl, drink the rest separately)

Lunch
Peanut Butter–Bacon Sandwich (page 179)
    1 cup celery and carrot sticks
    ¾ cup calcium-enriched V-8

Snack
4 oz sugar-free Jell-O

Dinner
3 to 4 oz fish of your choice (anything but fried; baked fish sticks are fine)
    1½ cups microwaved vegetables (combination of broccoli, carrots, and cauliflower, or your choice)
    ½ cup cooked brown rice (instant is fine), tossed with 1 Tbsp toasted slivered almonds and 1 tsp raisins

Evening Treat
Peanut Butter–Stuffed Dates (page 191)
    1,457 calories, 71 g protein, 187 g carbohydrates, 57 g fat, 12 g saturated fat, 25 g monounsaturated fat, 33 g fiber, 2,028 mg sodium, 845 mg calcium

DAY 20: SATURDAY

Breakfast
Peanut Butter Maple Syrup Waffles (page 202)
    1 cup fat-free milk, plain or in café latte

Lunch
1 frozen microwaveable bean burrito (about 260 calories and 6 to 8 g fat; Amy's Bean and Rice Burrito is a good choice)
    ½ cup raw vegetable of your choice (such as broccoli florets or baby carrots)

Snack
1 peach, 2 plums, or other fruit of your choice

Dinner
3 oz rotisserie chicken breast (about ½ small breast) from supermarket, skin removed
    ⅓ cup coleslaw (store-bought is fine)
    Salad: 3 cups greens, 1½ cups chopped vegetables of your choice with 2 Tbsp reduced-calorie olive- or canola-oil-based dressing

Evening Treat
Peanut Butter Ice Cream (page 190)
    1,517 calories, 79 g protein, 186 g carbohydrates, 57 g fat, 13 g saturated fat, 25 g monounsaturated fat, 24 g fiber, 1,949 mg sodium, 884 mg calcium

DAY 21: SUNDAY

Breakfast
Peanut Butter English Muffin Melt (page 190)
    1 cup fat-free milk, plain or in café latte

Lunch
1 cup lentil, black bean, or split pea soup (canned is fine)
simmered with ½ cup chopped broccoli, carrots or cauliflower and 2 cups fresh spinach (or ½ cup frozen)
    1 slice whole wheat bread

Snack
1 piece fruit of your choice

Dinner
Chicken Kebabs with Chinese Peanut Sauce (page 170)
    ½ cup brown rice (instant is fine)
    2 cups mushrooms, zucchini, onions, broccoli, or other
broiled vegetables of your choice: Brush with mix of 2
tsp reduced-sodium soy sauce; 1½ tsp olive, canola, or
peanut oil; and ½ tsp lemon juice. Broil at the same time
as the kebabs. Optional: Sprinkle with chopped parsley or
cilantro.

Evening Treat
Orange Creamsicle: In a blender, whip ¾ cup calcium-
enriched orange juice, ¼ cup fat-free milk, ½ tsp vanilla
extract, ¼ cup fat-free vanilla frozen yogurt, and 2 ice
cubes.

    1,511 calories, 81 g protein, 205 g carbohydrates, 50 g
fat, 10 g saturated fat, 23 g monounsaturated fat, 28 g
fiber, 3,777 mg sodium, 991 mg calcium

DAY 22: MONDAY

Breakfast
Peanut Butter Oatmeal (page 192)

Lunch
Salad: 2 cups mixed salad greens, ½ cup canned kidney beans rinsed and drained) and a small chopped pear or apple with 2 tsp extra-virgin olive oil, 2 tsp balsamic vinegar, ¼ tsp dried basil, and a sprinkle of garlic powder
     1 slice multigrain bread

Snack
¾ cup tomato juice

Dinner
Stir-fry 2 oz lean pork tenderloin in a nonstick pan with ½ cup each snow peas, broccoli florets, and slivered red bell peppers in 1 tsp peanut oil. Season with 1 Tbsp low-sodium soy sauce and 1 tsp Asian five-spice powder.
     ½ cup cooked brown rice (instant is fine)

Evening Treat
Peanut Butter–Banana Yogurt "Pudding" (page 193)
     1,500 calories, 76 g protein, 199 g carbohydrates, 55 g fat, 10 g saturated fat, 26 g monounsaturated fat, 37 g fiber, 1,993 mg sodium, 808 mg calcium

DAY 23: TUESDAY

Breakfast
1 cup Multi-Bran Chex with ½ cup frozen blueberries and 1 cup fat-free milk (if this is too much milk for your bowl, drink the rest separately)

Lunch
Veggie pita: Toss 1 cup salad greens, ¼ cup shredded carrots, ¼ cup shredded red cabbage, ⅛ avocado cut in chunks, and 1 Tbsp chopped peanuts with 1 Tbsp reduced fat olive- or canola-oil-based dressing. Stuff into a small whole wheat pita pocket.

1 cup fat-free plain yogurt

Snack
Peanut Butter Apple Slices (page 193)

Dinner
Sauté 2 oz thinly sliced lean eye of round beef in a non-stick pan with 1 small sliced yellow onion, 1 large sliced portabella mushroom, and 1 minced clove garlic in 1 tsp olive oil

5 microwaved asparagus spears

1 small baked sweet potato dusted with pumpkin pie spice

Evening Treat
Peanut Butter–Frosted Energy Bar (page 194)

1,535 calories, 73 g protein, 218 g carbohydrates, 55 g fat, 11 g saturated fat, 28 g monounsaturated fat, 34 g fiber, 1,493 mg sodium, 890 mg calcium

DAY 24: WEDNESDAY

Breakfast
Peanut Butter Breakfast Shake (page 194)

Lunch
1 cup instant black bean soup
 ½ cup raw broccoli florets
 ½ cup grapes

Snack
1 cup calcium-enriched orange juice

Dinner
3 oz broiled salmon
 ½ cup cooked whole wheat couscous
 1 cup frozen baby brussels sprouts and 1 cup frozen yellow squash, microwaved and topped with 1 Tbsp olive oil

Evening Treat
Peanut Butter English Muffin Melt (page 190)
 1,536 calories, 78 g protein, 195 g carbohydrates, 60 g fat, 11 g saturated fat, 28 g monounsaturated fat, 36 g fiber, 1,708 mg sodium, 988 mg calcium

DAY 25: THURSDAY

Breakfast
1 egg (or ¼ cup egg substitute) scrambled in a nonstick pan with ¼ cup each chopped green bell pepper and onions (frozen is fine) in 1 tsp canola oil, and salt and pepper to taste

2 clementine oranges or 1 orange
Whole grain or oat bran toasted English muffin

Lunch

Open-face tomato melt: Top 1 slice whole wheat bread with 1 thick slice fresh tomato and 1 slice reduced-fat Cheddar cheese. Broil in toaster oven until cheese melts.
1 medium banana

Snack

Peanut Butter–Stuffed Celery (page 183)

Dinner

Cook 1 cup dry whole wheat macaroni, then top with 1 cup low-fat mushroom-and-pepper pasta sauce. Add 12 large steamed shrimp (buy them presteamed at the seafood counter) and 2 Tbsp grated Parmesan cheese.
2 cups salad greens with 1 Tbsp reduced-calorie dressing

Evening Treat

Peanut Butter Sundae (page 192)
1,534 calories, 72 g protein, 184 g carbohydrate, 61 g fat, 11 g saturated fat, 28 g monounsaturated fat, 29 g fiber, 1,230 mg sodium, 698 mg calcium

DAY 26: FRIDAY

Breakfast

Peanut Butter–Strawberry Waffles (page 191)

Lunch

Salad: 2 cups baby spinach, ¼ cup sliced red onion, 5 grape tomatoes, and 4 oz flaked white water-packed tuna tossed with 1 Tbsp reduced-fat dressing and seasoned to taste with pepper and salt

1 medium orange

Snack
whole wheat cinnamon graham crackers

Kiwifruit

Dinner
Sauté ½ cup sliced yellow onion and 4 oz diced chicken breast (Perdue Short Cuts are fine) in 2 tsp olive oil. Stir into 2 cups cooked wild rice. Top with ½ Tbsp toasted chopped pecans.

1 cup microwaved fresh or frozen carrot slices

Evening Treat
Peanut Butter Sundae (page 192)

1,524 calories, 72 g protein, 184 g carbohydrates, 61 g fat, 11 g saturated fat, 28 g monounsaturated fat, 29 g fiber, 1,230 mg sodium, 698 mg calcium

DAY 27: SATURDAY

Breakfast
Peanut Butter French Toast (page 199)

½ cup strawberries

1 cup fat-free milk

Lunch
Veggie burger on whole grain bun with lettuce and tomato

1½ cups carrot and celery sticks

Snack
½ cup grapes or other fruit of your choice

Dinner
2 slices pizza with light cheese and extra veggies—
approximately ½ cup total veggies (each slice: ⅛ of 12"
pizza, about 140 calories per slice)
    Salad: 3 cups greens and 1 cup chopped vegetables of
your choice with 1½ Tbsp reduced-fat olive- or canola-
oil-based dressing
    8 oz light beer

Evening Treat
Peanut Butter Pudding in a Flash (page 180)
    1,554 calories, 67 g protein, 227 g carbohydrates, 51 g
fat, 12 g saturated fat, 20 g monounsaturated fat, 29 g
fiber, 2,572 mg sodium, 755 mg calcium

DAY 28: SUNDAY

Breakfast
½ large whole wheat or oat bran bagel with 2 oz lox and
1½ Tbsp reduced-fat cream cheese
    1 cup diced or 1 large wedge cantaloupe

Lunch
Peanut Butter–Bacon Sandwich (page 180)

Snack
1¼ cups raw vegetables of your choice (such as bell pepper strips, broccoli florets, or asparagus tips), dipped in ½
cup black bean dip (½ cup black beans mashed with ½
tsp olive oil and 2 Tbsp plain fat-free yogurt, and seasoned with a pinch of cumin, 1 Tbsp chopped fresh

cilantro or ½ tsp dried basil, and a dash of garlic powder; store-bought bean dip is fine)

¾ cup calcium-enriched V-8

Dinner
1 cup cooked whole wheat pasta with ⅓ cup marinara sauce and 1 Tbsp Parmesan cheese

1 heaping cup microwaved sugar snap peas (frozen are fine) with a dash of lemon and salt to taste

Evening Treat
S'More (page 200)

1 cup fat-free milk

1,551 calories, 80 g protein, 197 g carbohydrates, 57 g fat, 15 g saturated fat, 25 g monounsaturated fat, 34 g fiber, 3,835 mg sodium, 923 mg calcium

CHAPTER TWELVE

The Menu Plans for Men

Although women love it just as much, peanut butter has a reputation as a "guy food." So my colleagues and I thought, why not create a guys' version of the Peanut Butter Diet? That way, men can enjoy the same health benefits—a trimmer physique, a healthier heart, a lower risk of diabetes—while eating more of one of their all-time favorite foods!

Actually, the menu plans for men are very similar to those for women, with three noteworthy differences.

More peanut butter. Guys get three servings a day of 2 tablespoons each; women get two servings.

More calories. Each day's menu provides about 2,200 calories. By following the menu plans to the letter, the average man could lose about ½ pound a week, or 25 pounds over the course of a year. Just remember that if you want to slim down, you also need to accumulate 45 minutes of physical activity every day. That's your recommended daily amount of vitamin X, or "x-ercise." (For tips on increasing your activity level, check out chapter 15.)

More fiber. On the Peanut Butter Diet, men get about 35 grams of fiber a day—more than double the average intake. Research suggests that diets rich in fiber may reduce the risk of heart attack, stroke, and cancer. And in one study, every extra gram of fiber that people ate stopped their bodies from absorbing about 7 calories.

Despite these nutritional "extras," the guys' version of the menu plans coordinates quite well with the women's version. So if both you and your significant other want to try the Peanut Butter Diet, you can prepare meals and snacks together without a hitch.

DO THE DIET RIGHT

Just like the menu plans for women, those for guys get about 35 percent of their calories from fat—primarily the good-for-you monounsaturated fat found in peanut butter. Another 50 percent of calories come from carbohy-drates, and the rest—15 per-cent—from protein. The menu plans also provide for a super-nutritious nine servings of fruits and vegetables a day. These plant foods are packed with compounds

---

DID YOU KNOW . . .

Americans spend almost $800 million a year on peanut butter.

SOURCE: THE NATIONAL PEANUT BOARD

---

that appear to fight all sorts of health problems, includ-ing those so often associated with aging.

When a menu plan calls for one of the recipes in chap-ter 13, be sure that you use the ingredient amounts for men, as indicated in the recipe with asterisks (** means double the ingredient; *** means triple the ingredient). That way, you know you're getting enough calories over the course of a day.

If you prefer some menu plans over others or some peanut butter treats and recipes over others, feel free to make substitutions. Remember, though, that the replacement recipe should not exceed the original by more than about 25 calories.

One final note: Before you try the menu plans below, I do suggest that you read through "Supplements for Insurance" on page 104 and "A Word about Salt" on page 106. They have important information that can help you make the most of the Peanut Butter Diet.

Then get ready to indulge!

DAY 1: MONDAY

Breakfast
Peanut Butter Oatmeal (page 192)

Lunch
Bean burrito, restaurant or homemade (for homemade, combine an 8" tortilla, ½ cup beans, and 3 Tbsp salsa)

1 cup of red bell pepper strips, baby carrots, or other vegetable of your choice

¾ cup calcium-enriched V-8

Snack
1 cup fruit salad

Dinner
Chicken and vegetable stir-fry (2 cups vegetables, 4 oz chicken—a scant 1 cup): In a Chinese restaurant, ask for very little oil. A safer bet, calorie-wise: Sauté 1 tsp each minced ginger and garlic with 2 cups fresh or frozen vegetable mix containing broccoli in 1 tsp canola or peanut oil. Add your own chicken (precooked chicken like Perdue Short Cuts is fine). Season with teriyaki sauce.

1½ cups cooked brown rice (instant is fine)

Evening Treat
2 S'Mores (page 201)

2,223 calories, 105 g protein, 292 carbohydrates, 78 g fat, 18 g saturated fat, 34 g monounsaturated fat, 38 g fiber, 3,468 mg sodium, 911 mg calcium

DAY 2: TUESDAY

Breakfast
1 oz whole grain or bran cereal—should be 110 to 130 calories per ¾ to 1 cup, with at least 5 g fiber (Kellogg's Complete Wheat Bran Flakes and Kashi Good Friends are good choices)—with 1 small banana, sliced, and 1 cup fat-free milk (if this is too much milk for your bowl, drink the rest separately)

¾ cup calcium-fortified citrus juice

PB&J on Rye (page 202)

Lunch
Peanut Butter, Ham, and Pickle Sandwich (page 195)

1 cup cherry tomatoes and celery sticks

¾ cup calcium-enriched V-8

Snack
½ cup red bell pepper slices and 6 baked tortilla chips dipped in a ¼ cup bean dip (canned, or mash a heaping ¼ cup canned black beans with a dash of cumin, black pepper, and a few drops olive oil) and 2 to 4 Tbsp salsa. Optional: ½ tsp fresh cilantro.

Dinner
6 oz broiled fish of your choice

1 cup (about 8 spears) microwaved asparagus with a dash of lemon juice

1½ cups whole wheat couscous combined with 2 Tbsp raisins

Evening Treat
Peanut Butter Pudding in a Flash (page 197)

2,248 calories, 115 g protein, 326 g carbohydrates, 64 g fat, 13 g saturated fat, 27 g monounsaturated fat, 42 g fiber, 5,247 mg sodium, 991 mg calcium

DAY 3: WEDNESDAY

Breakfast
Mushroom scrambled eggs: In a nonstick pan, sauté ½ cup chopped mushrooms and 1 chopped scallion (optional) in 2 tsp olive or canola oil until wilted. Add 2 eggs and salt and pepper to taste. Serve with 2 toasted whole wheat or oat bran English muffins.

¾ cup calcium-enriched citrus juice

Lunch
Grilled chicken salad: In a restaurant, ask for dressing on the side and use the dip/spear method—dip your fork in the dressing, then spear a bite of salad. A safer bet, calorie-wise: Toss 3 cups greens with 1 Tbsp reduced-fat olive- or canola-oil-based dressing of your choice (Annie's Naturals Low-Fat Gingerly Vinaigrette is a good one), then add 6 oz grilled, skinless chicken strips (Perdue Short Cuts are fine).

1 slice whole wheat bread

Snack
Peanut Butter–Stuffed Celery (page 183)

Dinner

2 cups whole wheat spaghetti with ⅓ cup marinara sauce and 2 Tbsp Parmesan cheese

2 cups microwaved cauliflower, tossed with 2 tsp olive oil, 1 Tbsp Parmesan cheese, and a dash of lemon

Evening Treat

Peanut Butter Hot Chocolate (page 196)

2,163 calories, 143 g protein, 203 g carbohydrates, 98 g fat, 21 g saturated fat, 45 g monounsaturated fat, 36 g fiber, 2,545 mg sodium, 1,237 mg calcium

DAY 4: THURSDAY

Breakfast

Peanut Butter Breakfast Shake (page 194)

1 cup diced or 1 large wedge cantaloupe

2 slices rye toast, each spread with 1 tsp trans-free margarine

Lunch

Turkey sandwich: 4 oz sliced turkey breast with mustard, lettuce, and tomato on whole grain bread

Salad: 2 cups greens, 1 cup other vegetables, with 1 Tbsp reduced-fat olive- or canola-oil-based dressing

Snack

1 cup plain fat-free yogurt with 2 tsp maple syrup, a dash of vanilla extract, and 2 Tbsp trail mix

Dinner

⅔ cup Peanut Butter Creole Soup (page 197)

1 cup Cajun beans and rice: Use any mix, such as Uncle

Ben's Chef's Recipe, with about 210 calories per cup.
Add 1 cup mixed vegetables (such as frozen peas and carrots, thawed).

   ½ sliced cucumber with salt to taste

Evening Treat

Peanut Butter–Stuffed Dates (page 191)

   1 cup fat-free milk with 2 tsp Hershey's Syrup

   2,137 calories, 125 g protein, 271 g carbohydrates, 72 g fat, 15 g saturated fat, 31 g monounsaturated fat, 36 g fiber, 2,599 mg sodium, 1,586 mg calcium

DAY 5: FRIDAY

Breakfast

Peanut Butter–Frosted Energy Bar (page 194)

   1 cup fat-free milk, plain or in café latte

   2 tangerines or 1 large wedge cantaloupe

Lunch

⅔ cup Peanut Butter Creole Soup (page 197, or microwave last night's leftovers)

   Salad bar: At least 2 cups raw greens, 1½ cups other raw vegetables, 1 hard-boiled egg (or 3 Tbsp chopped egg), ½ cup beans (such as chickpeas or kidney beans), tossed with 2 Tbsp reduced-calorie olive- or canola-oil-based dressing

   2 slices whole wheat bread

Snack

Orange "soda": ¾ cup calcium-fortified citrus juice mixed with ½ cup seltzer

   Peanut Butter and Jelly Crackers (page 201)

Dinner

2 slices pizza—ask for light cheese and lots of extra veggies (each slice: ⅛ of 12" pizza, about 140 calories per slice, including ½ cup veggies per slice)
    ½ cup cucumber slices with salt to taste
    8 oz light beer

Evening Treat

½ cup strawberries or other berries topped with 1 cup low-fat vanilla yogurt and 1 Tbsp trail mix
    2,155 calories, 93 g protein, 283 g carbohydrates, 77 g fat, 18 g saturated fat, 32 g monounsaturated fat, 34 g fiber, 2,183 mg sodium, 1,692 mg calcium

DAY 6: SATURDAY

Breakfast

Peanut Butter Maple Syrup Waffles (page 202)
    1 cup fat-free milk, plain or in café latte

Lunch

Tuna salad: Combine a 6 oz can drained, water-packed, white albacore tuna with 4 tsp reduced-calorie mayonnaise, 1 tsp Dijon mustard, and 2 Tbsp finely chopped carrots and celery. Optional: 1 tsp chopped pickles.
    1½ cups baby carrots and red bell pepper strips
    ¾ cup calcium-enriched V-8
    ? slices whole wheat bread

Snack

Orange, pear, or other fruit of your choice
    1 cup vanilla low-fat yogurt

Dinner
Tahitian Chicken with Peanut Butter Mango Sauce (page 175), served over 1 cup cooked rice (preferably brown basmati)
½ cup cooked spinach

Evening Treat
1½"-thick slice angel food cake topped with 1½ cups coarsely mashed strawberries
Peanut Butter Pudding in a Flash (page 180)
2,796 calories, 129 g protein, 302 g carbohydrates, 5? g fat, 14 g saturated fat, 25 g monounsaturated fat, 28 g fiber, 2,931 mg sodium, 1,403 mg calcium

DAY 7: SUNDAY

Breakfast
Peanut Butter French Toast (page 200)
¾ cup calcium-enriched citrus juice

Lunch
Mediterranean salad: Combine ½ cup each chickpeas, chopped tomatoes, cucumbers, and red or green bell peppers. Mix with 2 Tbsp fresh basil (or 1 tsp dried), 2 tsp olive oil, and a scant tsp lemon juice. Add salt and pepper to taste.
2 slices crusty whole grain bread, each brushed with ¼ tsp olive oil and grilled or toasted

Snack
6 baked tortilla chips dipped in 2 to 4 Tbsp salsa

Dinner
Chicken Kebabs with Chinese Peanut Butter Sauce (page 170)
1 cup cooked brown rice (instant is fine)

Yogurt cucumber salad: Combine ¾ cup plain fat-free yogurt with ¼ cup finely chopped cucumbers, ½ tsp dried mint, and a dash of garlic powder or ¼ tsp fresh garlic.

Evening Treat

1 cup strawberries
    Peanut Butter Sundae (page 192)
    2,159 calories, 125 g protein, 258 g carbohydrates, 77 g fat, 19 g saturated fat, 34 g monounsaturated fat, 32 g fiber, 2,165 mg sodium, 1,331 mg calcium

DAY 8: MONDAY

Breakfast

1 oz whole grain or bran cereal—should be 110 to 130 calories per ¾ to 1 cup, with at least 5 g fiber (Kashi Go Lean and Barbara's Puffins are good choices)—with 1 small banana, sliced, and 1 cup fat-free milk (if this is too much milk for your bowl, drink the rest separately)

Lunch

Turkey-avocado bagel: Fill a 3- to 4-oz whole wheat or oat bran bagel with 4 oz sliced turkey, ¼ avocado, sliced, lettuce, and tomato slices
    ¾ cup calcium-enriched V-8
    1 cup fruit salad

Snack

2 small cookies (2½" diameter) of your choice
    1 cup instant hot chocolate

Dinner

Cold Peanut Butter Noodles (page 181)
    Spinach and carrot salad: Toss together 3 cups spinach

leaves, 1 carrot, grated, and 1 chopped scallion. Combine ½ tsp low-sodium soy sauce, ½ tsp honey, 1 tsp canola oil (for a blander flavor) or olive oil (for a stronger flavor), and ½ tsp lemon juice. Toss with the salad.

Evening Treat
Peanut Butter–Stuffed Celery (page 183)
   2,180 calories, 113 g protein, 297 g carbohydrates, 74 g fat, 15 g saturated fat, 35 g monounsaturated fat, 33 g fiber, 3,059 mg sodium, 1,150 mg calcium

DAY 9: TUESDAY

Breakfast
Scrambled egg sandwich: In a nonstick pan, scramble 1 egg and 1 egg white with ½ tsp canola or olive oil. Place between 2 slices whole wheat bread with 3 slices tomato.
   1 cup diced or 1 large wedge cantaloupe
   1 cup fat-free milk, plain or in café latte

Lunch
1½ cups lentil, split pea, or black bean soup (canned is fine)
   2 slices crusty whole grain bread
   Salad: 3 cups greens, 1 cup chopped vegetables, with 1½ Tbsp reduced-calorie olive- or canola-oil-based dressing
   ¾ cup calcium-enriched V-8

Snack
Peanut Butter Banana (page 203)

Dinner
Frozen dinner based on chicken—350 to 380 calories, 8 g fat (examples: Lean Cuisine Hearty Portions Chicken and Barbecue Sauce or Healthy Choice Country Breaded Chicken)

1 slice whole wheat bread dipped in 1 tsp olive oil
1 cup cherry tomatoes

Evening Treat

2 servings Angel Food Cake with Peanut Butter "Icing" (page 195)

2,239 calories, 102 g protein, 300 g carbohydrates, 80 g fat, 17 g saturated fat, 37 g monounsaturated fat, 40 g fiber, 3,896 mg sodium, 1,063 mg calcium

DAY 10: WEDNESDAY

Breakfast

Peanut Butter Oatmeal (page 192) (add 2 tsp maple syrup)

Lunch

Salad bar: 3 cups spinach with ½ cup tomato slices; ½ cup cauliflower or other vegetable of your choice; ½ cup chickpeas, kidney beans, or other beans; 1 hard-boiled egg (or 3 Tbsp chopped egg) and 2 Tbsp reduced-fat olive- or canola-oil-based dressing

¾ cup calcium-enriched V-8
1 ounce whole wheat crackers

Snack

1 small cookie (about 2½" diameter) of your choice
1 cup fat-free milk, plain or in café latte

Dinner

Sweet and Bacon-y Peanut Butter Muffins (page 176)

Salad: 3 cups Bibb lettuce, ½ cup chopped celery, 1 tangerine, sectioned, 1 chopped scallion and 1 Tbsp slivered almonds tossed with 1 Tbsp orange juice, 1 tsp olive oil, ½ tsp lemon juice, and salt and pepper to taste

Evening Treat
Peanut Butter Sundae (page 192) topped with ½ cup coarsely mashed fresh or frozen strawberries

2,176 calories, 96 g protein, 272 g carbohydrates, 91 g fat, 18 g saturated fat, 42 g monounsaturated fat, 37 g fiber, 3,117 mg sodium, 1,302 mg calcium

DAY 11: THURSDAY

Breakfast
2 mozzarella or string cheese sticks (for example, Polly-O or Sargento, about 70 calories apiece)
½ oz whole grain crackers
1 cup grapes

Lunch
Peanut Butter and Jelly Sandwich (page 168; use 3 Tbsp peanut butter)
1 cup red pepper slices dipped in ¼ cup plain fat-free yogurt mixed with a dash of garlic salt
Fruit "soda": ¾ cup fruit juice of your choice combined with ½ cup seltzer

Snack
3 Hershey's Kisses
3 Tbsp trail mix
1 cup fat-free milk

Dinner
Turkey chili: Sauté ⅓ lb ground turkey with chili seasoning and onions (optional). Combine with 2 cups chopped zucchini, 1 cup canned refried beans, and 1 cup canned or frozen corn. Add water as needed and heat through. (Serves 2; eat just half.)

1 cup cooked brown rice (instant is fine)
¾ cup calcium-enriched V-8
1 slice cornbread (2½" square)
Note: Reserve ½ cup corn for tomorrow's lunch

Evening Treat
Peanut Butter Pudding in a Flash (page 180; use 3 Tbsp peanut butter)

2,210 calories, 103 g protein, 274 g carbohydrates, 87 g fat, 24 g saturated fat, 36 g monounsaturated fat, 26 g fiber, 2,496 mg sodium, 1,351 mg calcium

DAY 12: FRIDAY

Breakfast
Peanut Butter Breakfast Shake (page 194)
1 cup grapes

Lunch
Corn, chicken, and bean salad: Combine ½ cup canned or frozen corn with ½ cup beans of your choice (chickpeas or white cannelloni work well), ½ cup chopped green or red bell peppers, ½ cup chopped or cherry tomatoes, 2 oz chopped chicken (a heaping ⅓ cup; Perdue Short Cuts are a good, quick choice). Toss with 2 Tbsp reduced-fat olive- or canola-oil-based dressing of your choice. Optional: 1 Tbsp fresh cilantro.
1 piece fruit of your choice

Snack
2 servings Peanut Butter and Jelly Crackers (page 201)

Dinner
6 to 8 oz broiled or steamed fish of your choice
1½ cups microwaved vegetables tossed with a dash of lemon and salt and pepper to taste

Four ½"-thick slices of polenta (buy premade polenta "logs"), each topped with ½ tsp Parmesan cheese and grilled in toaster oven according to polenta package directions (or use 2 large slices crusty whole grain bread)

Evening Treat
Orange Creamsicle: In a blender, whip ¾ cup calcium-enriched orange juice, ¼ cup fat-free milk, ½ tsp vanilla extract, ½ cup frozen vanilla fat-free yogurt, and 2 ice cubes.

2,167 calories, 121 mg protein, 260 g carbohydrates, 82 g fat, 16 g saturated fat, 38 g monounsaturated fat, 33 g fiber, 1,779 mg sodium, 1,107 mg calcium

DAY 13: SATURDAY

Breakfast
2 eggs, fried in 2 tsp olive or canola oil, with ⅔ cup cooked polenta (two 1½"-thick slices)
   1 orange or other fruit of your choice

Lunch
2 servings Peanut Butter, Bacon, and Cornbread Squares (page 188)
   1½ cups red bell pepper strips and celery sticks
   1 cup fat-free milk

Snack
1 apple or other fruit of your choice

Dinner
1 cup low-sodium tomato soup simmered with ½ cup peas, chopped carrots, or other vegetable of your choice
   6 oz. rotisserie chicken breast from supermarket, skin removed

Baked potato topped with ½ cup chopped broccoli and ¼ cup plain fat-free yogurt

Evening Treat
Peanut Butter Sundae (page 192)

2,216 calories, 104 g protein, 246 g carbohydrates, 90 g fat, 19 g saturated fat, 37 g monounsaturated fat, 30 g fiber, 2,384 mg sodium, 1,030 mg calcium

DAY 14: SUNDAY

Breakfast
Peanut Butter Cinnamon Toast (page 186)

1 cup fat-free milk, plain or in café latte
1 cup sliced strawberries or any other fruit of your choice

Lunch
Tuna salad sandwich on whole wheat. To make tuna salad: Combine one 6-oz can drained, water-packed, white albacore tuna with 4 tsp reduced-calorie mayonnaise, 1 tsp Dijon mustard, and 2 Tbsp chopped celery. Optional: 2 tsp chopped pickles.

1½ cups baby carrots and red bell pepper strips

Snack
¾ cup calcium-enriched V-8

12 baked tortilla chips dipped in ¼ cup guacamole (store-bought is fine)

Dinner
Peanut Butter Island Shrimp (page 172)

1 cup cooked brown basmati rice (or instant brown rice)
1 cup microwaved sugar snap peas (frozen are fine) dressed with ½ tsp olive oil and a dash of lemon juice

Evening Treat
3 small cookies (about 2½" diameter) such as Chips Ahoy soft cookies (great microwaved)
Peanut Butter Hot Chocolate (page 196)
2,198 calories, 133 g protein, 238 g carbohydrates, 89 g fat, 19 g saturated fat, 41 g monounsaturated fat, 33 g fiber, 3,853 mg sodium, 1,359 mg calcium

DAY 15: MONDAY

Breakfast
Peanut Butter–Frosted Energy Bar (page 194)
1 cup fat-free milk, plain or in café latte
7 dried apricot halves or 2 Tbsp raisins

Lunch
Peanut Butter and Jelly Sandwich (page 168)
½ cup celery sticks
Fruit "soda": ¾ cup fruit juice of your choice, ½ cup seltzer

Snack
1 cup fruit salad topped with ¼ cup low-fat vanilla yogurt

Dinner
Bean bruschetta: Heat ½ cup cannelloni beans. Remove from heat and mash coarsely with 1 tsp chopped fresh basil (or ¾ tsp dried) and ½ tsp olive oil. Grill 3 slices crusty whole grain bread, each brushed with ½ tsp olive oil. Spread with bean mixture and top with 1 tsp Parmesan cheese.
Greek salad: Toss together ¼ cup cannelini beans, 3 cups greens, 8 cherry tomatoes or 1 medium chopped

tomato, ½ cup chopped cucumber, ¼ cup green or red bell peppers, sliced and ½ tsp dried oregano. Toss with 2 Tbsp reduced-calorie canola-oil-based or olive-oil-based dressing. Top with 3 Tbsp crumbled feta cheese and 2 olives.

Evening Treat

1 cup fat-free milk, plain or in café Latte
S'More (page 201)
Note: Prepare Gingered Peanut Butter–Carrot Spread (page 185) for next day
2,228 calories, 85 g protein, 291g carbohydrates, 92 g fat, 20 g saturated fat, 45 g monounsaturated fat, 39 g fiber, 2,180 mg sodium, 1,524 mg calcium

DAY 16: TUESDAY

Breakfast

1 oz whole grain or bran cereal—should be 110 to 130 calories per ¾ to 1 cup, with at least 5 g fiber (Kellogg's Complete Wheat Bran Flakes and Kashi Good Friends are good choices)—with 1 small banana, sliced, and 1 cup fat-free milk (if this is too much milk for your bowl, drink the rest separately)
¾ cup calcium-fortified citrus juice
1 slice whole wheat toast spread with 1 tsp trans-free margarine

Lunch

Turkey sandwich: 4 oz sliced turkey breast with mustard, lettuce, and tomato on whole grain bread
1 cup red bell pepper strips dipped in ½ cup Gingered Peanut Butter–Carrot Spread (page 185)

Snack
1 cup fruit salad
  Peanut Butter–Stuffed Dates (page 191)

Dinner
Veggie burger (Gardenburger, Amy's California Veggie
Burger, and Boca Burger are all good choices) on whole
grain bun with lettuce, 3 slices tomato, ¼ avocado, and 2
Tbsp crumbled feta cheese
  6 baked tortilla chips dipped in ¼ cup guacamole
(store-bought is fine)

Evening Treat
Peanut Butter Hot Chocolate (page 196)
  2,162 calories, 123 g protein, 257 g carbohydrates,
87 g fat, 19 g saturated fat, 38 g monounsaturated fat, 42
g fiber, 2,703 mg sodium, 1,129 mg calcium

DAY 17: WEDNESDAY

Breakfast
Whole wheat or oat bran English muffin, cut in half, and
toasted, spread with ½ cup Gingered Peanut Butter–
Carrot Spread (page 185)
  1 cup fat-free milk, plain or in café latte
  1 cup diced or 1 large wedge cantaloupe

Lunch
1½ cups lentil, split pea, or black bean soup (canned or instant is fine)
  2 slices crusty whole grain bread
  Salad: 3 cups greens, 1 cup chopped vegetables, and 2
Tbsp reduced-fat olive- or canola-oil-based dressing

Snack
¾ cup calcium-enriched citrus juice
   2 Tbsp trail mix

Dinner
"Kitchen sink" pasta: To 1½ cups cooked whole wheat ziti or other short pasta, add 1 cup diced tomatoes, 2 olives, ¾ cup cooked, skinless chicken (Perdue Short Cuts are fine), ½ cup microwaved vegetable of your choice (such as frozen broccoli or snow peas). Toss with 4 tsp olive oil and season with 1½ Tbsp chopped fresh basil (or 1 tsp dried). Add salt and pepper to taste.

Evening Treat
Peanut Butter Ice Cream (page 190)
   2,249 calories, 110 g protein, 269 g carbohydrates, 81 g fat, 14 g saturated fat, 38 g monounsaturated fat, 34 g fiber, 3,835 mg sodium, 1,252 mg calcium

DAY 18: THURSDAY

Breakfast
Peanut Butter Bagel (page 203)
   1 cup fruit salad
   1 cup fat-free milk, plain or in café latte

Lunch
Grilled chicken salad: In a restaurant, ask for dressing on the side and use the dip-spear method—dip your fork in the dressing, then spear a piece of salad. A safer bet, calorie-wise: Toss 3 cups greens with 6 oz grilled, skinless chicken strips (Perdue Short Cuts are fine) and 1 Tbsp reduced-fat olive- or canola-oil-based dressing of your choice.
   1 orange or other fruit of your choice

Snack
1 small cookie (2½" diameter) of your choice
   1 cup fat-free milk, plain or in café latte

Dinner
Homemade burrito: Heat a 6" to 8" tortilla (preferably whole wheat) and fill with ½ cup canned refried beans, 1 or 2 leaves chopped lettuce, 2 to 4 Tbsp salsa, and ¼ cup guacamole (store-bought is fine).

Mexican grilled vegetables: Skewer 6 regular mushrooms and 1 zucchini (about 5") cut in diagonal slices. Brush with a combo of 2 tsp olive oil, ½ tsp chili powder, 1 tsp lime juice, and ½ clove crushed garlic (optional). Grill (or broil 5" from the broiler) for 5 minutes, turn, brush again, and grill 5 minutes longer, or until softened.

Evening Treat
S'Mores (page 200)
   2,224 calories, 130 g protein, 248 g carbohydrates, 91 g fat, 21 g saturated fat, 42 g monounsaturated fat, 31 g fiber, 3, 073 mg sodium, 998 mg calcium

DAY 19: FRIDAY

Breakfast
1 oz whole grain or bran cereal—should be 110 to 130 calories per ¾ to 1 cup, with at least 5 g fiber (Kellogg's Complete Wheat Bran Flakes and Kashi Good Friends are good choices)—with 1 small banana, sliced, and 1 cup fat-free milk (if this is too much milk for your bowl, drink the rest separately)
   ¾ cup calcium-fortified citrus juice
   PB&J on Rye (page 201)

Lunch
Peanut Butter–Bacon Sandwich (page 179)
   1 cup celery and carrot sticks
   ¾ cup calcium-enriched V-8

Snack
4 oz sugar-free Jell-O

Dinner
6 to 8 oz fish of your choice (anything but fried; baked fish sticks are fine)
   1½ cups microwaved vegetables (combination of broccoli, cauliflower, and carrots or your choice)
   1 cup cooked brown rice (instant is fine), tossed with 2 Tbsp toasted slivered almonds and 2 tsp raisins

Evening Treat
Peanut Butter–Stuffed Dates (page 191)
   2,230 calories, 106 g protein, 275 g carbohydrates, 91 g fat, 18 g saturated fat, 41 g monounsaturated fat, 41 g fiber, 2,457 mg sodium, 948 mg calcium

DAY 20: SATURDAY

Breakfast
Peanut Butter Maple Syrup Waffles (page 202)
   1 cup fat-free or 1% milk, plain or in café latte
   ¾ cup calcium-enriched citrus juice

Lunch
1 frozen, microwaveable bean burrito (about 260 calories and 6 to 8 g fat; Amy's Bean and Rice Burrito is a good choice)
   ½ cup raw vegetable of your choice (such as broccoli florets, or baby carrots)

6 baked tortilla chips dipped in 2 Tbsp guacamole (store-bought is fine)

Snack
1 peach, 2 plums, or other fruit of your choice

Dinner
6 oz rotisserie chicken breast from supermarket, skin removed

⅓ cup coleslaw (store-bought is fine)

Salad: 3 cups greens, 1½ cups chopped vegetables of your choice with 2 Tbsp reduced-calorie olive- or canola-oil-based dressing

1 slice crusty whole grain bread dipped in 1 tsp olive oil

Evening Treat
2 servings Peanut Butter Sundae (page 192)

2,161 calories, 127 g protein, 198 g carbohydrates, 89 g fat, 20 g saturated fat, 33 g monounsaturated fat, 24 g fiber, 2,505 mg sodium, 1,485 mg calcium

DAY 21: SUNDAY

Breakfast
Peanut Butter English Muffin Melt (page 190)

1 cup fat-free milk, plain or in café latte

Lunch
1½ cups lentil, black bean, or split pea soup (canned is fine) simmered with ½ cup chopped broccoli, carrots, or cauliflower and 2 cups fresh spinach (or ½ cup frozen)

2 slices whole wheat bread

Snack

1 piece fruit of your choice
   3 Tbsp trail mix

Dinner

Chicken Kebabs with Chinese Peanut Sauce (page 170)
(double entire recipe)
   1½ cups cooked brown rice (instant is fine)
   2 cups broiled vegetables of your choice (such as
mushrooms, zucchini, onions, or broccoli): Brush with
mix of 2 tsp reduced-sodium soy sauce; 1½ tsp olive,
canola, or peanut oil; ½ tsp lemon juice. Broil at the same
time as the kebabs. Optional: Sprinkle with chopped
parsley or cilantro.

Evening Treat

Orange Creamsicle: In a blender, whip ¾ cup calcium-
enriched orange juice, ¼ cup fat-free milk, ½ tsp vanilla
extract, ¼ cup fat-free vanilla frozen yogurt, and 2 ice
cubes.

   2,224 calories, 117 g protein, 283 g carbohydrates,
79 g fat, 16 g saturated fat, 35 g monounsaturated fat,
36 g fiber, 5,227 mg sodium, 1,071 mg calcium

DAY 22: MONDAY

Breakfast

Peanut Butter Oatmeal (page 192)

Lunch

Salad: 2 cups mixed salad greens, 1 cup canned kidney
beans (rinsed and drained) and a small chopped pear or
apple with 2 tsp extra-virgin olive oil, 2 tsp balsamic
vinegar, ¼ tsp dried basil, and a sprinkle of garlic powder
   2 slices multigrain bread

Snack
¾ cup calcium-enriched V-8

Dinner
Stir-fry 2 oz lean pork tenderloin in nonstick pan with ½ cup each snow peas, broccoli florets, and slivered red bell peppers in 1 tsp peanut oil. Season with 1 Tbsp low-sodium soy sauce and 1 tsp Asian five-spice powder.
    1 cup cooked brown rice (instant is fine)

Evening Treat
2 servings Peanut Butter–Banana Yogurt "Pudding" (page 193)
    2,498 calories, 115 g protein, 360 g carbohydrates, 78 g fat, 15 g saturated fat, 34 g monounsaturated fat, 43 g fiber, 3,296 mg sodium, 1,384 mg calcium

DAY 23: TUESDAY

Breakfast
2 cups Multi-Bran Chex with ½ cup frozen blueberries and 1 cup fat-free milk (if this is too much milk for your bowl, drink the rest separately)

Lunch
Veggie pita: Toss 1 cup salad greens, ¼ cup shredded carrots, ¼ cup shredded red cabbage, ⅛ avocado cut in chunks, and 1 Tbsp chopped peanuts with 1 Tbsp reduced-fat olive- or canola-oil-based dressing. Stuff into small whole wheat pita pocket.
    1 cup fat-free plain yogurt

Snack
Peanut Butter Apple Slices (page 193)

Dinner

Sauté 6 oz thinly sliced lean eye of round beef in a non-stick pan with 1 small sliced yellow onion, 1 large sliced portabella mushroom, and 1 minced clove garlic in 1 tsp olive oil.

5 microwaved asparagus spears

1 large baked sweet potato dusted with pumpkin pie spice

Evening Treat

Peanut Butter–Frosted Energy Bar (page 194)

2,468 calories, 117 g protein, 341 g carbohydrates, 109 g fat, 23 g saturated fat, 38 g monounsaturated fat, 35 g fiber, 2,290 mg sodium, 1,098 mg calcium

DAY 24: WEDNESDAY

Breakfast

Peanut Butter Breakfast Shake (page 194)

Lunch

1 cup instant black bean soup
    ½ cup raw broccoli florets
    ½ cup grapes

Snack

1 cup calcium-enriched orange juice

Dinner

6 oz broiled salmon
    1½ cups cooked whole wheat couscous
    1 cup frozen baby brussels sprouts and 1 cup frozen yellow squash, microwaved and topped with 1 Tbsp olive oil

Evening Treat
Peanut Butter English Muffin Melt (page 190)
  2,223 calories, 112 g protein, 285 g carbohydrates, 82 g fat, 14 g saturated fat, 37 g monounsaturated fat, 40 g fiber, 2,185 mg sodium, 938 mg calcium

DAY 25: THURSDAY

Breakfast
1 egg (or ¼ cup egg substitute) scrambled in a nonstick pan with ¼ cup each chopped green bell pepper and onions (frozen is fine) in 1 tsp canola oil and salt and pepper to taste
  2 clementine oranges or 1 orange
  1½ whole grain English muffins, toasted

Lunch
Open-face tomato melt: Top 2 slices whole wheat bread with 1 thick slice fresh tomato and 1 slice reduced-fat Cheddar cheese on each. Broil in a toaster oven until cheese melts.
  1 medium banana

Snack
Peanut Butter–Stuffed Celery (page 183)

Dinner
Cook 2 cups dry whole wheat macaroni, then top with 1 cup low-fat mushroom-and-pepper pasta sauce. Add 24 large steamed shrimp (buy them presteamed at the seafood counter) and 2 Tbsp Parmesan cheese.
  2 cups salad greens with 1 Tbsp reduced-fat dressing

Evening Treat
Peanut Butter–Stuffed Dates (page 191)

2,674 calories, 132 g protein, 367 g carbohydrates, 90 g fat, 22 g saturated fat, 36 g monounsaturated fat, 31 g fiber, 3,082 mg sodium, 710 mg calcium

DAY 26: FRIDAY

Breakfast
Peanut Butter Strawberry Waffles (page 191)

Lunch
Salad: 2 cups baby spinach, ¼ cup sliced red onion, 5 grape tomatoes, and 4 oz flaked white water-packed tuna tossed with 1 Tbsp reduced-fat dressing and seasoned to taste with pepper and salt

1 medium orange

Snack
Peanut Butter and Jelly Crackers (page 200)

Kiwifruit

Dinner
Sauté ½ cup sliced yellow onion and 4 oz diced chicken breast (Perdue Short Cuts are fine) in 2 tsp olive oil. Stir into 2 cups cooked wild rice. Top with ½ Tbsp toasted chopped pecans.

1 cup microwaved fresh or frozen carrot slices

Evening Treat
Peanut Butter Sundae (page 192)

2,246 calories, 116 g protein, 274 g carbohydrates, 86 g fat, 12 g saturated fat, 33 g monounsaturated fat, 40 g fiber, 3,106 mg sodium, 424 mg calcium

DAY 27: SATURDAY

Breakfast
Peanut Butter French Toast (page 199)
  ½ cup strawberries
  1 cup fat-free milk
  1 cup calcium-enriched citrus juice

Lunch
Veggie burger on whole grain bun with lettuce, tomato, and ¼ sliced avocado
  1½ cups carrot and celery sticks
  12 baked tortilla chips

Snack
1 cup grapes or 1 other fruit of your choice
  Peanut Butter and Jelly Crackers (page 200)

Dinner
2 slices pizza with light cheese and extra veggies—about ½ cup total veggies (each slice: ⅛ of 12" pizza, about 140 calories per slice)
  Salad: 3 cups greens and 1 cup chopped vegetables of your choice with 1½ Tbsp reduced-fat olive- or canola-oil-based dressing
  1 large slice crusty whole grain bread dipped in 2 tsp olive oil
  8 oz light beer

Evening Treat
Peanut Butter Pudding in a Flash (page 180)
  2,177 calories, 80 g protein, 297 g carbohydrates, 86 g fat, 18 g saturated fat, 40 g monounsaturated fat, 38 g fiber, 2,822 mg sodium, 756 mg calcium

DAY 28: SUNDAY

Breakfast
1 large whole wheat or oat bran bagel with 3 oz lox and 3 Tbsp reduced-fat cream cheese
   1 cup diced or 1 large wedge cantaloupe

Lunch
Peanut Butter–Bacon Sandwich (page 179)

Snack
1¼ cups raw vegetables of your choice (such as bell pepper strips, broccoli florets, or asparagus spears) dipped in ½ cup black bean dip (½ cup black beans mashed with ½ tsp olive oil and 2 Tbsp plain fat-free yogurt, and seasoned with a pinch of cumin, 1 Tbsp chopped fresh cilantro or ½ tsp dried basil, and a dash of garlic powder; store-bought bean dip is fine)
   ¾ cup calcium-enriched V-8

Dinner
1½ cups cooked whole wheat pasta with ⅓ cup marinara sauce and 2 Tbsp Parmesan cheese
   1 heaping cup microwaved sugar snap peas (frozen are fine) with a dash of lemon and salt to taste

Evening Treat
2 S'Mores (page 200)
   1 cup fat-free milk
   2,203 calories, 108 g protein, 278 g carbohydrates, 84 g fat, 24 g saturated fat, 36 g monounsaturated fat, 42 g fiber, 5,038 mg sodium, 1,062 mg calcium

CHAPTER THIRTEEN

The Recipes

You love peanut butter. You'd love to eat peanut butter and lose weight. So you're sure to love this collection of 50 fabulous recipes that make the Peanut Butter Diet easy—and absolutely scrumptious.

My colleagues at *Prevention* magazine taste-tested scores of peanut butter creations in the Rodale Test Kitchen, under the direction of *Prevention*'s food editor, Regina Ragone, R.D., and test kitchen manager JoAnn Brader. Only the yummiest, easiest dishes made it into this book.

Some of the recipes may seem absurdly obvious, like the one for a Peanut Butter and Jelly Sandwich (page 168). Why on earth am I telling people how to make PB&J? For starters, I suspect that anyone who has been living in the Land of Low Fat for quite a few years may need a little help in overcoming any fear of eating peanut butter. Seeing the directions for an old favorite on paper just might do the trick. What's more, since the recipe lists a specific amount for each ingredient, you'll be able to make your sandwich with the confidence that you are not going to break your calorie bank and put on weight.

Many of the recipes are super-quick: You take some peanut butter and mix it with this or spread it on that. Voilà! You're good to go.

A handful of recipes may seem a bit more complex. *Do not be scared off by them.* They may have more than two or three ingredients, but they're here because they're amazingly delicious and truly easy, usually calling for a combination of several convenience foods and some seasonings.

Not all of the recipes appear in the menu plans in chapters 11 and 12. Some are so unique and appetizing that I just had to pass them along! If you spot a recipe that makes your mouth water but isn't featured in any of the menus, you may substitute it for another recipe as long as it has roughly the same number of calories as the original. When swapping recipes, try not to increase your day's calorie intake by more than 25.

PING-PONG PORTION CONTROL

Before you start sampling our peanut butter creations, get out your Ping-Pong ball—remember it from chapter 8?—and put it somewhere on your kitchen counter where it will stay in plain sight and won't roll away. I keep mine in a wooden bowl with my bananas.

By now you know that a Ping-Pong ball is almost precisely the same size as 2 tablespoons of peanut butter, the amount in a serving of most of the recipes. If you haven't already done so, I strongly suggest that you go through the process of measuring out exactly 2 tablespoons of peanut butter with a measuring spoon. That way, you can see what the amount looks like and how closely it matches your Ping-Pong ball.

From then on, when you need 2 tablespoons of peanut butter, you can use a regular kitchen teaspoon—the kind you use to stir your coffee—to scoop out a glob that's the same size as the ball. It's so much simpler than measuring.

Just keep yourself honest. For the Peanut Butter Diet to work, especially if you want to lose weight, you *must* stick with the 2-tablespoon-per-serving portion. As healthy as peanut butter can be, it's very high in calories. Going even a little over-board could backfire and make you gain weight. Nei-ther you nor I want that to

> **DID YOU KNOW . . .**
>
> Americans eat enough peanut butter in a year to make more than 10 billion peanut butter and jelly sandwiches.
>
> SOURCE: THE NATIONAL PEANUT BOARD

happen. (And it's just what some experts are betting will happen! Wouldn't you love to prove them wrong?)

Of course, some of the recipes that make several servings call for as much as ½ cup of peanut butter at a time. For that amount, your best bet may be to use a measuring cup. If you're pressed for time, remember that ½ cup equals 8 tablespoons, or four Ping-Pong balls. Likewise, ¼ cup equals 4 tablespoons, or two Ping-Pong balls.

SPECIAL INSTRUCTIONS FOR MEN

Because the Peanut Butter Diet provides 2,200 calories a day for men, compared with 1,500 calories a day for women, some of the recipes have been "guy-sized" to in-clude slightly larger quantities of specific ingredients. These variations are noted with asterisks: ** is your cue to double the amount of the ingredient; *** means you should triple it.

My colleagues and I hope that you love these recipes as much as we do. You'll see just how versatile and very, very satisfying peanut butter can be!

CREAMY OR CRUNCHY: IT'S UP TO YOU

You'll notice that some of the recipes specify creamy or crunchy peanut butter. This means that when we prepared the recipe in the Rodale Test Kitchen, we decided that we liked it best with one kind of peanut butter or the other. But if you prefer creamy over crunchy, or vice versa, go right ahead and use your favorite.

Whether we used creamy or crunchy, we did find that emulsified peanut butter—the kind in which the oil doesn't rise to the top—was easiest to work with.

Peanut Butter and Jelly Sandwich

If there's one single food that seems most American, a lot of people would vote for the good old PB&J. It's sad that so many of us gave up eating this all-time favorite before we learned that its monounsaturated fat was actually good for our hearts. We know you know how to make one of these without a recipe, but we hope that actually seeing the directions and ingredient amounts written down will encourage you to overcome the last residue of unnecessary Fear of Peanut Butter.

- 2 slices whole wheat bread
- 2 Tbsp peanut butter
- 1 Tbsp grape jelly (or other jelly or jam of your choice)

Spread one slice of the bread with the peanut butter. Spread the jelly over the peanut butter, then top with the second slice of bread. Slice in half and enjoy!

MAKES I SERVING

PER SERVING: 371 calories,

While writing this book, guess who I discovered eats a peanut butter and jelly sandwich almost every day for lunch? The author of *Prevention*'s "Supplement News" column, nutrition expert Densie Webb, R.D., Ph.D.

13 g protein, 44 g carbohydrates, 18 g fat, 4 g saturated
fat, 8 g monounsaturated fat, 0 mg cholesterol, 6 g fiber,
436 mg sodium

Fluffer-Nutter

We knew you'd be looking for this kiddie classic at least
once. Nothing in a Fluffer-nutter is nutritionally redeem-
ing but the peanut butter, so we substituted cracked wheat
bread for the traditional white bread for more crunch and
fiber.

    2 slices cracked wheat bread
    2 Tbsp peanut butter
    2 Tbsp marshmallow cream

Spread 1 slice of bread with 2 Tbsp peanut butter, then
top with 2 Tbsp marshmallow cream. Put the bread slices
together, then cut in half.

MAKES 1 SERVING

PER SERVING: 386 calories, 12 g protein, 48 g carbohydrates, 18 g fat, 3.3 g saturated fat, 8 g monounsaturated
fat, 1 mg cholesterol, 3 g fiber, 434 mg sodium

Peanut Butter, Chicken, and Pineapple Pita

This sandwich is a snap to prepare, thanks to the strips of
precooked chicken available in the poultry section of the
supermarket.

    1 cup chopped, cooked chicken breast
    ½ cup canned, crushed, unsweetened pineapple,
        drained
    ⅓ cup chopped celery
    ⅓ cup canned, chopped water chestnuts, drained

⅓ cup chopped red bell pepper
½ cup creamy peanut butter
2 Tbsp light teriyaki sauce
1½ Tbsp lemon juice
½ tsp ground ginger
½ tsp onion powder
⅛ tsp dry mustard
4 6" pita rounds (oat bran or whole wheat)
8 lettuce leaves
1 cup broccoli sprouts

> Most people slice their sandwiches on the diagonal, to wind up with two triangle-shaped halves. But when I was a child, I insisted that my sandwiches be sliced horizontally, so that each half formed a rectangle. I still do.

Combine the chicken, pineapple, celery, water chestnuts, and pepper in a large bowl. In a small bowl, mix the peanut butter, teriyaki sauce, lemon juice, ginger, onion powder, and mustard. Mix the peanut butter dressing into the chicken salad. Line each pita pocket (½ of the pita round) with one lettuce leaf and fill with broccoli sprouts and chicken salad.

MAKES 4 SERVINGS

PER SERVING: 456 calories, 30 g protein, 53 g carbohydrates, 21 g fat, 4 g saturated fat, 8 g monounsaturated fat, 35 mg cholesterol, 3 g fiber, 545 mg sodium

Chicken Kebabs with Chinese Peanut Butter Sauce

The lovely peanut butter sauce for these kebabs also makes a great dip for crudités.

1 lb boneless, skinless chicken breast
2 Tbsp low-sodium soy sauce
1½ tsp vegetable oil

1 tsp packed brown sugar
¼ tsp ground ginger
1 clove garlic, crushed
1 cup Chinese Peanut Butter Sauce (page 181)

Cut the chicken into ¾" pieces. (For easier cutting, partially freeze the chicken for about 1 hour.) In a glass bowl, mix the chicken with the soy sauce, oil, brown sugar, ginger, and garlic. Cover and refrigerate for at least 2 hours, stirring occasionally. Soak 8 bamboo skewers in water for at least 30 minutes before using to prevent burning.

Set the oven to broil. Remove the chicken and reserve the marinade. Thread 4 or 5 chicken pieces on each skewer. Brush the chicken with the reserved marinade.

Broil the chicken about 4" from the heat for 4 to 5 minutes. Turn; brush with more of the marinade. Broil 4 to 5 minutes longer, or until the chicken is no longer pink in the center. Discard any remaining marinade. Serve the chicken with ¼ cup peanut butter sauce per serving.

MAKES 4 SERVINGS
PER SERVING: 374 calories, 35 g protein, 10 g carbohydrates, 23 g fat, 4 g saturated fat, 11 g monounsaturated fat, 66 mg cholesterol, 2 g fiber, 743 mg sodium

Peanut Butter Pasta with Cucumber and Spicy Peanut Sauce

Look for English cucumbers, which are seedless. Sliced red peppers can be purchased in the produce department.

1 cup creamy peanut butter
¼ cup soy sauce
¼ cup lemon juice

3 cloves garlic, minced
1 tsp red-pepper flakes
1 tsp sugar
1½ cups hot water
16 oz whole wheat pasta
2 cucumbers, peeled, seeded, and cut diagonally into
    ⅛" slices
1 cup chopped scallions
1 cup thinly sliced red bell peppers (1" long)

In a blender, combine the peanut butter, soy sauce, lemon juice, garlic, red-pepper flakes, sugar, and water until smooth. In a pot of boiling salted water, cook the pasta until just tender; transfer to a colander and rinse briefly under cold water. Drain well. In a large bowl, toss the pasta with the peanut sauce, cucumbers, scallions, and peppers. Serve immediately or at room temperature.
MAKES 8 SERVINGS
PER SERVING: 412 calories, 17 g protein, 55 g carbohydrates, 17 g fat, 3 g saturated fat, 8 g monounsaturated fat, 0 mg cholesterol, 4 g fiber, 812 mg sodium

Peanut Butter Island Shrimp

Time-savers: Make sure you buy the cleaned, peeled shrimp that seafood departments now offer. Keep frozen shrimp on hand for when you need a last-minute dinner.

1 tsp sesame oil
1 Tbsp peanut oil
1¼ cups chopped onion
1 tsp chopped fresh ginger
2 tomatoes, peeled and chopped
1 tsp salt
1¼ tsp red-pepper flakes

1 bay leaf
1 can (8 oz) tomato sauce
1½ lb raw shrimp, peeled
¾ cup hot water
¾ cup crunchy peanut butter
Chopped cilantro
3 cups hot, cooked Jasmine rice

Heat the sesame and peanut oils in a large skillet; add the onion and ginger, and sauté over low heat until tender, but not browned. Add the tomatoes, salt, red-pepper flakes, bay leaf, and tomato sauce. Cover and simmer for 15 minutes. Add the shrimp. Blend the hot water with the peanut butter and add to the mixture. Cover and simmer for 10 minutes longer. Remove the bay leaf. Garnish with the cilantro and serve over the rice.

MAKES 6 SERVINGS
PER SERVING: 492 calories, 35 g protein, 44 g carbohydrates, 20 g fat, 4 g saturated fat, 9 g monounsaturated fat, 175 mg cholesterol, 5 g fiber, 919 mg sodium

Note: If you don't have fresh tomatoes, use ½ cup canned, diced tomatoes.

Curried Peanut Butter Soup

This soup is fabulous—well worth a little extra prep time. When *Prevention* staffers tasted it, everybody raved! Start a dinner party with this soup, and your guests will want the recipe.

¾ cup shredded carrot
½ cup chopped onion
½ cup chopped celery
1 Tbsp butter
1 Tbsp peanut oil

2 Tbsp all-purpose flour
1 tsp curry powder
¼ tsp salt
3½ cups reduced-sodium chicken broth
2 tsp Worcestershire sauce
¾ cup crunchy peanut butter

In a 2-quart saucepan, cook the carrot, onion, and celery in the butter and oil until tender, about 10 minutes.

Blend in the flour, curry powder, and salt. Add the chicken broth and Worcestershire sauce. Cook, stirring, until thickened and bubbly.

Reduce the heat; add the peanut butter and stir until melted.

Serve hot with condiments (see note).

MAKES 6 SERVINGS

PER SERVING: 259 calories, 10 g protein, 13 g carbohydrates, 20 g fat, 4 g saturated fat, 9 g monounsaturated fat, 5 mg cholesterol, 3 g fiber, 559 mg sodium

Note: To make this a completely vegetarian soup, use reduced-sodium vegetable broth instead of chicken broth.

Sprinkle your soup with any of the following condiments: chopped dried pineapple, shredded coconut, chopped scallions, chopped peanuts, raisins, curry powder.

Creamy Carolina Peanut Soup

To intensify the peanut flavor and lower the saturated fat in this recipe, substitute peanut oil for the olive oil and butter.

1 small onion, chopped
1 rib celery, chopped
1 Tbsp butter

1 Tbsp olive oil
¼ cup all-purpose flour
4 cups chicken broth
1 cup crunchy peanut butter
1 cup 2% milk

Combine the onion, celery, butter, and oil in a 3-quart saucepan. Cook over medium-low heat for about 10 minutes. Stir in the flour, then gradually stir in the broth. Bring to a boil. Reduce the heat and simmer for about 15 minutes. Add the peanut butter. Puree the mixture in a food processor or blender and return to the pan. Over low heat, stir in the milk to the desired temperature.

MAKES 8 SERVINGS
PER SERVING: 260 calories, 11 g protein, 13 g carbohydrates, 20 g fat, 5 g saturated fat, 9 g monounsaturated fat, 6 mg cholesterol, 3 g fiber, 426 mg sodium

Tahitian Chicken with Peanut Butter Mango Sauce

This was one of our favorite peanut butter recipes! Definitely good enough for company. If you want to cut down on the number of ingredients, omit the honey and the mustard and just use 1 Tbsp honey mustard.

Chicken
3 boneless, skinless chicken breast halves
2 Tbsp peanut oil
¼ tsp salt
⅛ tsp pepper
Sauce
¾ cup mango chutney
¾ cup crunchy peanut butter
1 tsp curry powder
½ tsp Dijon mustard

1 clove garlic, crushed
1 Tbsp honey
2 Tbsp oil
2–4 Tbsp hot water

To make the chicken: Preheat the broiler or grill. Cut each chicken breast half in two, making 6 pieces. Brush the chicken with the oil and sprinkle with the salt and pepper. Cook about 4" from the heat for about 8 minutes each side, or until cooked through.

> The size of the average boneless, skinless chicken breast half is about 6 ounces. Since the size of a healthy serving of meat is 3 ounces, about the size of a deck of cards, you can plan on getting 2 servings per chicken breast half.

To make the sauce: Coarsely chop any pieces of fruit in the chutney and return to the liquid. Combine the chutney with the peanut butter, curry powder, mustard, garlic, honey, and oil. Add water to thin and heat until melted.

> Never tried mango chutney? It's delicious. You'll often find it in the Ethnic food section at your supermarket. And you'll also be able to use it in our Peanut Butter, Bacon, and Cornbread Squares on page 188.

Spread the sauce over the grilled chicken.

MAKES 6 SERVINGS
PER SERVING: 459 calories, 34 g protein, 33 g carbohydrates, 22 g fat, 4 g saturated fat, 10 g monounsaturated fat, 66 mg cholesterol, 2 g fiber, 666 mg sodium

Sweet and Bacon-y Peanut Butter Dinner Muffins

When *Prevention* staffers first heard the ingredients for this recipe, most didn't expect to like the result. But these sandwiches ended up being one of our most delicious surprises. Experiment with different flavors of English muffins such as honey wheat or sourdough.

1 tsp vegetable oil
12 slices (about 8 oz) Canadian bacon
½ cup crunchy peanut butter
¼ cup orange marmalade
4 English muffins, split and lightly toasted
2 tsp Dijon mustard
2 Tbsp light mayonnaise
Chopped chives (optional)

Heat the oil in a 10" skillet over medium heat. Add the Canadian bacon and cook for several minutes, or until hot and beginning to brown. Meanwhile, combine the peanut butter and marmalade in a small bowl. Spread on 1 side of each muffin. Top with 3 slices of Canadian bacon. Combine the mustard and mayonnaise in a small bowl, then spread over the bacon. Sprinkle with the chives (if using). Cover with the remaining muffin halves.

MAKES 4 SANDWICHES

PER SERVING: 447 calories, 20 g protein, 46 g carbohydrates, 21 g fat, 3 g saturated fat, 8 g monounsaturated fat, 22 mg cholesterol, 3 g fiber, 1,096 mg sodium

> *Prevention's* alternative medicine editor, Sara Altshul, tried cutting these sandwiches into bite-size pieces to serve as hors d'oeuvres. They were a big hit!

Note: To reduce the sodium in this sandwich, cut the amount of Canadian bacon in half.

Hot Peanut Butter Milk

This creamy drink met with serious skepticism from some testers, until they tried it! If you love peanut butter, you'll love this comforting concoction.

1 cup fat-free milk
2 Tbsp creamy peanut butter
1 Tbsp honey
Ground cinnamon or grated nutmeg

In a small saucepan, heat the milk and peanut butter over low heat, stirring continuously. When the milk is hot and the peanut butter has melted and blended completely, stir in the honey to taste.

Remove the pan from the heat. With a small whisk, briskly stir the milk to form a light froth. Pour the milk into a large, heated mug and lightly dust with the cinnamon or nutmeg before serving.

MAKES I SERVING

PER SERVING: 342 calories, 16 g protein, 36 g carbohydrates, 16 g fat, 3 g saturated fat, 8 g monounsaturated fat, 4 mg cholesterol, 2 g fiber, 280 mg sodium

> For a festive touch, use a whole cinnamon stick as a stirrer.

Peanutty Apple Sandwiches

Peanut butter and apples are a classic combo, but this sandwich gives them extra pizzazz. Experiment with some of the newer varieties of apples, such as Pink Lady, Gala, and Ginger Crisps.

½ cup crunchy peanut butter
¼ cup apricot preserves
¼ tsp ground mustard
4 cinnamon raisin English muffins, toasted
½ medium apple, thinly sliced
4 lettuce leaves

Stir together the peanut butter, preserves, and mustard. Spread on 4 muffin halves.

Place the apple slices on the peanut butter mixture; top with the lettuce leaves and the remaining 4 muffin halves.

MAKES 4 SERVINGS

PER SERVING: 400 calories, 12 g protein, 52 g carbohydrates, 17 g fat, 3 g saturated fat, 8 g monounsaturated fat, 0 mg cholesterol, 4 g fiber, 517 mg sodium

Peanut Butter–Bacon Sandwiches

Vegetarian? No problem. There are a variety of tasty, meatless, baconlike strips available in the supermarket, which you can use as substitutes.

¼ cup creamy or crunchy peanut butter
2 slices crisp-cooked bacon, crumbled
4 slices raisin bread

In a small bowl, mix the peanut butter and bacon; spread on 2 bread slices. Top with the remaining bread.

MAKES 2 SERVINGS

PER SERVING: 425 calories, 15 g protein, 47 g carbohydrates, 22 g fat, 4 g saturated fat, 9 g monounsaturated fat, 5 mg cholesterol, 7 g fiber, 406 mg sodium

---

Have you discovered precooked bacon yet? You'll never want the mess of making bacon from scratch again. Look for this wonderful convenience food in boxes at the bacon counter. Just pop as many slices as you need in the microwave for 10 seconds each. They come out crispy and delicious.

Peanut Butter Pudding in a Flash

Almost nothing is quicker than making this ultra-rich snack using single-serving fat-free pudding cups. It's really sensational.

   1 single-serving container (4 oz) of prepared, fat-free
      refrigerated pudding of your choice (chocolate,
      vanilla, or tapioca)**
   2 Tbsp crunchy peanut butter

Place the peanut butter in a microwaveable dessert dish. Microwave on high for about 1 minute, or until melted. Pour the pudding into the peanut butter, and stir until mixed through.

MAKES 1 SERVING

PER SERVING FOR WOMEN: 290 calories, 10 g protein, 30 g carbohydrates, 16 g fat, 3 g saturated fat, 8 g monounsaturated fat, 0 mg cholesterol, 2 g fiber, 386 mg sodium

PER SERVING FOR MEN: 390 calories, 12 g protein, 53 g carbohydrate, 16 g fat, 3 g saturated fat, 8 g mono-

---

If you'd rather make 4 servings of peanut butter pudding at a time, here's an alternate recipe that's quick and delicious.

2 cups cold fat-free milk
½ cup crunchy peanut butter
1 pkg (3¾ oz) instant pudding (any flavor)

Pour the milk into a medium bowl. Add the peanut butter and pudding mix and beat slowly just until well-mixed, about 1 minute. Pour into serving dishes. Let stand for about 5 minutes to set.

MAKES 4 SERVINGS

PER SERVING: 326 calories, 12 g protein, 36 g carbohydrates, 16 g fat, 3 g saturated fat, 8 g monounsaturated fat, 2 mg cholesterol, 2 g fiber, 566 mg sodium

unsaturated fat, 0 mg cholesterol, 2 g fiber, 616 mg
sodium

> Have you ever wondered what tapioca is? It's a starchy substance
> extracted from the root of the cassava plant and formed into a
> pellet, which is called pearl tapioca. Pearl tapioca is used mainly to
> make puddings.

Chinese Peanut Butter Sauce

We tested many peanut butter sauces. Happily, the one we
liked the best was also the easiest to make! It's great over
noodles (see Cold Peanut Butter Noodles, below) or even
as a salad dressing.

¼ cup crunchy peanut
butter
2 tsp reduced-sodium soy
sauce
½ tsp sugar
⅛ tsp garlic salt
5 Tbsp water

> It pays to use reduced-sodium
> soy sauce. It can have half as
> much salt as regular soy sauce.

In a medium bowl, combine the peanut butter, soy sauce,
sugar, garlic salt, and 1 Tbsp of the water. Gradually add
the remaining 4 Tbsp water and stir until evenly blended.
MAKES 2 SERVINGS
PER SERVING: 196 calories, 8 g protein, 8 g carbohydrates, 16 g fat, 3 g saturated fat, 8 g monounsaturated
fat, 0 mg cholesterol, 2 g fiber, TK g sodium

Cold Peanut Butter Noodles

This recipe uses the Chinese Peanut Butter Sauce
(above) to great advantage. This one was suggested by our

assistant food editor, Sherry Kiser, because it's one of her favorite quick and easy dinners. She serves it with spinach salad.

> This dish may be served hot, but Sherry likes it best at room temperature.

    1 cup cooked whole wheat or buckwheat (soba)
        noodles
    ½ cup chopped cucumber
    ¼ cup Chinese Peanut Butter Sauce
    1 chopped scallion (optional)

In a medium bowl, combine the noodles and cucumber, then top with the sauce and scallions (if using).

> For an instant garnish, keep a can or jar of chopped peanuts in the fridge. Many of the recipes in the Peanut Butter Diet can be topped with a sprinkle of chopped peanuts for an extra-special touch.

MAKES I SERVING

PER SERVING: 535 calories, 24 g protein, 64 g carbohydrates, 24 g fat, 5 g saturated fat, 11 g mono-unsaturated fat, 0 mg cholesterol, 4 g fiber, 666 g sodium

Peanut Butter–Bacon Spread

Did you know that 1 strip of bacon has only 48 calories and 4 grams of fat? Its addition to this dish makes eating vegetables a pleasure.

    6 Tbsp creamy peanut butter
    ½ tsp Worcestershire sauce
    2 Tbsp chili sauce
    4 slices bacon, cooked and crumbled

In a medium bowl, blend the peanut butter, Worcestershire sauce, and chili sauce; add the bacon. Spread on crackers.

MAKES 3 SERVINGS

PER SERVING: 248 calories, 11 g protein, 9 g carbohydrates, 20 g fat, 5 g saturated fat, 10 g monounsaturated fat, 7 mg cholesterol, 2 g fiber, 430 mg sodium

Peanut Butter–Stuffed Celery

Celery stuffed with plain peanut butter is a well-loved staple—and a great way to get one more serving of veggies. But you'll be amazed how much adult kick just a little horseradish adds to this childhood snack—without adding any calories!

   ¼ cup creamy or crunchy peanut butter**
   2 Tbsp horseradish**
   2 ribs celery**

In a small bowl, mix the peanut butter and horseradish. If necessary, add a small amount of water to soften the mixture. Spread half of the mixture in each celery rib. Wrap the stuffed celery in plastic or aluminum foil to chill.

MAKES 2 SERVINGS

PER SERVING FOR WOMEN: 197 calories, 8 g protein, 9 g carbohydrates, 16 g fat, 3 g saturated fat, 8 g monounsaturated fat, 0 mg cholesterol, 3 g fiber, 271 mg sodium

PER SERVING FOR MEN: 394 calories, 16 g protein, 18 g carbohydrates, 32 g fat, 6 g saturated fat, 16 g monounsaturated fat, 0 mg cholesterol, 6 g fiber, 542 mg sodium

> Bottled horseradish, found in the dairy case, is available in white (preserved in vinegar) and red (preserved in beet juice). We prefer the white for this recipe.

The Ultimate Peanut Butter–Stuffed Celery

Here's another zesty version of the classic peanut butter snack. Try fennel as a refreshing alternative to the celery.

> ¾ cup crunchy peanut butter, at room temperature
> 1 pkg (3 oz) fat-free cream cheese, softened
> 1 Tbsp Worcestershire sauce, or to taste
> Tabasco sauce, to taste
> ¼ cup finely chopped scallions
> 6 ribs celery, trimmed and chilled

In a medium bowl, stir together the peanut butter, cream cheese, Worcestershire sauce, and Tabasco until blended. Fold in the scallions.

With a knife, spread a dollop of the mixture down the hollow of each celery rib. Arrange the ribs on a tray or plate and serve immediately.

MAKES 6 SERVINGS

PER SERVING: 221 calories, 13 g protein, 9 g carbohydrates, 16 g fat, 3 g saturated fat, 8 g monounsaturated fat, 0 mg cholesterol, 3 g fiber, 317 mg sodium

Hot Maple Peanut Drink

For the best possible flavor, use real maple syrup rather than maple-flavored syrup. If you don't need your drink sweet, cut back to 1 Tbsp of maple syrup and save 55 calories.

> 2 Tbsp creamy peanut butter
> 2 Tbsp maple syrup
> 1 cup milk
> Dash of ground cinnamon or ground nutmeg

In a saucepan, beat together the peanut butter, syrup, milk, and cinnamon or nutmeg. Heat until steaming. Serve in a mug with a cinnamon stick stirrer.

MAKES 1 SERVING

PER SERVING: 384 calories, 16 g protein, 48 g carbohydrates, 16 g fat, 3 g saturated fat, 8 g monounsaturated fat, 4 mg cholesterol, 2 g fiber, 320 mg sodium

Peanut Butter Ice Cream Shake

To make a lower-calorie version of this treat, cut the chocolate syrup and frozen yogurt amounts in half.

  2 Tbsp creamy peanut butter
  1 Tbsp chocolate syrup
  1 cup fat-free vanilla frozen yogurt or ice cream

Combine the peanut butter, chocolate syrup, and yogurt or ice cream in a blender until smooth and thick. Serve in chilled glass.

MAKES 1 SERVING

PER SERVING: 430 calories, 14 g protein, 60 g carbohydrates, 16 g fat, 3 g saturated fat, 8 g monounsaturated fat, 0 mg cholesterol, 2 g fiber, 303 mg sodium

Gingered Peanut Butter–Carrot Spread

This adult peanut butter spread is a great way to eat your carrots. Use some spread to fill whole wheat pitas, and make extra for dipping the next day. We like golden raisins for a change of pace.

Think of peanut butter as an "incentive food." Adding it to fruit or veggies that you might not otherwise eat is a smart move.

   2 carrots, peeled and grated
   ⅓ cup raisins, chopped
   ½ cup crunchy peanut butter
   ¼ cup fat-free mayonnaise
   ½ tsp ground ginger

In a medium bowl, combine the carrots, raisins, peanut
butter, mayonnaise, and ginger.

MAKES 4 SERVINGS

PER SERVING: 327 calories, 11 g protein, 35 g carbohydrates, 18 g fat, 3 g saturated fat, 8 g monounsaturated
fat, 0 mg cholesterol, 5 g fiber, 455 mg sodium

The two most common types of raisins available are dark and
golden. Both are made from Thompson seedless grapes. The dark
raisins are sun-dried for several weeks, while the moister, plumper
golden has been treated with sulfur dioxide and dried with artifi-
cial heat. Both are rich in iron.

Peanut Butter Cinnamon Toast

You may find that you like this just as well with less sugar
than we call for. Great—you'll save some calories!

   2 Tbsp creamy or chunky peanut butter
   1 Tbsp brown sugar
   ½ tsp ground cinnamon
   1 slice whole grain bread

In a small bowl, blend the peanut butter, brown sugar, and
cinnamon. Toast the bread and immediately spread with
the peanut butter mixture. Allow to melt.

MAKES 1 SERVING

PER SERVING: 304 calories, 10 g protein, 32 g carbohydrates, 17 g fat, 3 g saturated fat, 8 g monounsaturated fat, 0 mg cholesterol, 5 g fiber, 316 mg sodium

Peanut Butter Bread Pudding with Raisins

This hot breakfast pudding has just the right amount of sweetness to make a perfect Sunday brunch treat. If you have any leftovers, use them chilled with a small dollop of whipped cream for a delightful dessert.

    6 slices raisin bread, cut into 1" cubes
    1¾ cups milk
    4 large eggs
    ¾ cup creamy peanut butter
    3 Tbsp brown sugar
    1 tsp vanilla extract
    1 tsp grated fresh or ¼ tsp dried orange peel

Coat a 9" × 9" baking pan with cooking spray. Add the bread cubes and set aside.

In a blender, combine the milk, eggs, peanut butter, brown sugar, vanilla, and orange peel. Process until smooth. Pour the mixture evenly over the bread cubes in the baking pan, saturating them. Cover with foil and refrigerate overnight.

Preheat the oven to 350°F. Remove the foil and bake for about 35 minutes, or until lightly browned and puffed.

MAKES 6 SERVINGS

PER SERVING: 410 calories, 17 g protein, 37 g carbohydrates, 23 g fat, 6 g saturated fat, 9 g monounsaturated fat, 152 mg cholesterol, 5 g fiber, 308 mg sodium

Peanut Butter, Bacon, and Cornbread Squares

Use the fat-free packaged corn muffin mix sold in the baking aisle of your supermarket for the cornbread squares in this recipe.

> 2 2" cornbread squares
> ¼ cup creamy peanut butter
> 2 slices cooked bacon
> 2 Tbsp mango chutney

Cut the cornbread squares in half and spread each bottom half with 2 Tbsp of the peanut butter. Top with 1 slice of crumbled bacon and the remaining half of the cornbread. Heat in a toaster oven until warmed through.

MAKES 2 SERVINGS

PER SERVING: 384 calories, 12 g protein, 39 g carbohydrates, 22 g fat, 4 g saturated fat, 8 g monounsaturated fat, 0 mg cholesterol, 4 g fiber, 736 mg sodium

> You can save time by using precooked bacon that you crisp in the microwave.

Peanut Butter Baked Apples

These apples will remind you of the caramel-dipped apples we enjoyed as kids.

> 2 large baking apples
> ¼ cup creamy peanut butter
> 2½ Tbsp maple syrup
> ¼ cup water
> ½ tsp ground cinnamon

Core the apples. Peel the upper halves and place in a shallow baking dish. In a medium bowl, mix the peanut butter and ½ Tbsp of the maple syrup until blended. Spoon into the centers of the apples. In a small bowl, combine the remaining 2 Tbsp maple syrup with the water and cinnamon. Pour over the apples.

Cover loosely with waxed paper. Microwave on high for 4 to 5 minutes, or until fork-tender. Let stand for 3 minutes before serving.

MAKES 2 SERVINGS

PER SERVING: 380 calories, 8 g protein, 57 g carbohydrates, 17 g fat, 3 g saturated fat, 8 g monounsaturated fat, 0 mg cholesterol, 5 g fiber, 198 mg sodium

Peanut Butter "Sweets"

Bake these sweet potatoes the night before to take to work for a satisfying lunch. Reheat a potato half in the cafeteria microwave, then spread with peanut butter.

2 medium sweet potatoes, baked
½ cup crunchy peanut butter
Dash of ground cinnamon

Cut the hot sweet potatoes in half. Spread each half with 2 Tbsp of the peanut butter and sprinkle with cinnamon.

MAKES 4 SERVINGS

PER SERVING: 258 calories, 9 g protein, 23 g carbohydrates, 16 g fat, 3 g saturated fat, 8 g monounsaturated fat, 0 mg cholesterol, 3 g fiber, 165 mg sodium

Peanut Butter Ice Cream

The richness of the peanut butter makes ordinary fat-free ice cream or fat-free frozen yogurt a decadent treat. For a smooth texture, use creamy peanut butter, and for a chunky texture, use the crunchy variety.

    ¾ cup fat-free vanilla or chocolate frozen yogurt or
        ice cream, slightly softened
    2 Tbsp creamy or crunchy peanut butter

Combine the yogurt or ice cream and the peanut butter in a bowl and mix thoroughly. Cover the bowl and place it in the freezer until firm.

MAKES I SERVING

PER SERVING: 340 calories, 12 g protein, 38 g carbohydrates, 16 g fat, 3 g saturated fat, 8 g monounsaturated fat, 0 mg cholesterol, 2 g fiber, 261 mg sodium

Peanut Butter
English Muffin Melt

Why is it that when peanut butter melts, it offers a whole new dimension of satisfaction?

    ½ whole wheat English muffin
    2 Tbsp creamy or crunchy peanut butter

Toast the muffin to desired doneness and spread with the peanut butter.

MAKES I SERVING

PER SERVING: 253 calories, 10 g protein, 20 g carbohydrates, 16 g fat, 3 g saturated fat, 8 g monounsaturated fat, 0 mg cholesterol, 3 g fiber, 243 mg sodium

Peanut Butter-Stuffed Dates

Dried dates are available year-round and are sold packaged, either pitted or unpitted. Dates are a good source of protein and iron.

  4 large dried pitted dates
  2 Tbsp creamy peanut butter

Slit the dates in half and press the centers with a teaspoon to make room for the peanut butter. Spoon the peanut butter into the dates.

MAKES I SERVING

PER SERVING: 279 calories, 9 g protein, 31 g carbohydrates, 16 g fat, 3 g saturated fat, 8 g monounsaturated fat, 0 mg cholesterol, 5 g fiber, 154 mg sodium

Peanut Butter–Strawberry Waffles

This topping can be used on any of the wide variety of healthy frozen waffles (such as soy and flax) and French toast now available in the supermarket. For a change, try mashed blueberries or bananas in place of the strawberries.

  2 whole grain waffles
  2 Tbsp creamy peanut butter
  ½ cup frozen strawberries, thawed and mashed

Toast the waffles, then spread with the peanut butter. Top with the strawberries.

MAKES I SERVING

PER SERVING: 434 calories, 14 g protein, 45 g carbohydrates, 24 g fat, 3 g saturated fat, 8 g monounsaturated fat, 0 mg cholesterol, 8 g fiber, 594 mg sodium

Peanut Butter Sundae

Find the lowest-calorie fat-free frozen yogurt or ice cream you can. Use vanilla or chocolate or be more creative—it's up to you. When you top it with melted peanut butter, you'll feel like you're eating something sinful.

2 Tbsp creamy peanut butter
½ cup fat-free frozen yogurt or ice cream (any flavor)

Place the peanut butter in a small microwaveable dish. Heat on high for about 1 minute, or until melted. Drizzle over the frozen yogurt.

MAKES I SERVING

PER SERVING: 268 calories, 11 g protein, 25 g carbohydrates, 16 g fat, 3 g saturated fat, 8 g monounsaturated fat, 0 mg cholesterol, 3 g fiber, 218 mg sodium

Peanut Butter Oatmeal

Have trouble getting your kids to eat breakfast? Here's one that both you and the kids will love.

¼ cup dry old-fashioned oats**
½ cup fat-free milk**
4 dried apricot halves, cut into quarters
2 Tbsp crunchy peanut butter
¼ tsp ground cinnamon

In a microwaveable bowl, combine the oats, milk, and apricots. Microwave on high for 3 minutes. Stir in the peanut butter and cinnamon.

MAKES I SERVING

PER SERVING FOR WOMEN: 413 calories, 17 g protein, 53 g

carbohydrates, 18 g fat, 3 g saturated fat, 8 g monounsaturated fat, 2 mg cholesterol, 6 g fiber, 221 mg sodium
PER SERVING FOR MEN: 751 calories, 39 g protein, 105 g carbohydrates, 22 g fat, 5 g saturated fat, 11 g monounsaturated fat, 8 mg cholesterol, 8 g fiber, 415 mg sodium

Peanut Butter–Banana Yogurt "Pudding"

This is one of the quickest treats you can make. For added pizzazz, try chocolate-flavored yogurt.

>   2 Tbsp creamy peanut butter
>   ¾ cup fat-free plain yogurt
>   ½ banana, sliced

In a microwaveable dessert dish, heat the peanut butter for about 1 minute, or until melted. Stir in the yogurt and top with the banana.
MAKES I SERVING
PER SERVING: 388 calories, 19 g protein, 46 g carbohydrates, 17 g fat, 3 g saturated fat, 8 g monounsaturated fat, 3 mg cholesterol, 4 g fiber, 285 mg sodium

Peanut Butter Apple Slices

The old adage about an apple a day keeping the doctor away is now more true than ever. A study conducted by researchers from Finland's National Public Health Institute in Helsinki found that the flavonoids from apples played a critical role in decreasing the risk of lung cancer.

>   1 red or golden Delicious apple, sliced into
>   8 segments
>   2 Tbsp creamy peanut butter

Spread the peanut butter on the apple slices and fan them out on a small plate.

MAKES I SERVING

PER SERVING: 269 calories, 8 g protein, 28 g carbohydrates, 16 g fat, 3 g saturated fat, 8 g monounsaturated fat, 0 mg cholesterol, 5 g fiber, 154 mg sodium

Peanut Butter–Frosted Energy Bar

Everyone has her favorite granola or energy bar. Especially if you pick one with a high fiber count, it makes a great snack. When you add peanut butter, it's irresistible.

   1 fat-free date-almond granola bar
   2 Tbsp creamy peanut butter

Spread the peanut butter on the granola bar.

MAKES I SERVING

PER SERVING: 314 calories, 10 g protein, 26 g carbohydrates, 21 g fat, 5 g saturated fat, 9 g monounsaturated fat, 0 mg cholesterol, 3 g fiber, 232 mg sodium

Peanut Butter Breakfast Shake

If you really want to be decadent, try low-fat or fat-free chocolate milk in place of the regular fat-free milk.

   1 cup fat-free milk
   1 small, ripe banana
   2 Tbsp toasted wheat germ (see note)
   2 Tbsp creamy peanut butter

Combine the milk, banana, wheat germ, and peanut butter in a blender and blend until smooth.

MAKES I SERVING
PER SERVING: 433 calories, 22 g protein, 52 g carbohydrates, 18 g fat, 4 g saturated fat, 8 g monounsaturated
fat, 4 mg cholesterol, 6 g fiber, 281 mg sodium
  Note: Use wheat germ only on Day 24.

Peanut Butter, Ham, and Pickle Sandwich

Hundreds of readers wrote to tell us their favorite food to
eat with peanut butter was pickles! Here is our version,
with a little twist.

  2 Tbsp creamy or crunchy peanut butter
  2 slices whole grain bread
  2 Tbsp pickle relish
  1 slice (½ oz) low-fat deli ham

Spread the peanut butter on 1 slice of the bread. Spread
the pickle relish on top of the peanut butter and top with
the remaining slice of bread.

MAKES I SERVING
PER SERVING: 370 calories,
16 g protein, 39 g carbo-
hydrates, 19 g fat, 3 g saturated fat, 8 g monoun-
saturated fat, 4 mg cholesterol, 8 g fiber, 880 mg
sodium

> What's the best pickle to go
> with peanut butter—a sweet
> gherkin or a kosher dill? Our
> readers are just about evenly
> divided. (I vote for the sweet
> gherkin!)

Angel Food Cake with Peanut Butter "Icing"

This quick topping can perk up any low-fat dessert. We
like it on angel food cake or frozen yogurt. Be sure to use
the icing while it is still hot.

    2 Tbsp creamy peanut butter
    1 Tbsp apricot preserves
    1 Tbsp 1% milk
    1 slice angel food cake 1½" thick

Combine the peanut butter and preserves in a small microwaveable bowl. Microwave on high for 30 to 40 seconds, or until melted. Add the milk and stir until smooth. Spread on the cake.

MAKES 1 SERVING

PER SERVING: 395 calories, 13 g protein, 53 g carbohydrates, 17 g fat, 3 g saturated fat, 8 g monounsaturated fat, 2 mg cholesterol, 2 g fiber, 304 mg sodium

Peanut Butter Hot Chocolate

This drink is so easy and unbelievably delicious. Look for calcium-fortified cocoa mix for an extra hit of nutrition.

    2 Tbsp creamy peanut butter
    6 oz boiling water
    1 pkg (0.55 oz) sugar-free hot cocoa mix

Spoon the peanut butter into a mug. Pour about 2 Tbsp of the water onto the peanut butter and stir until it forms a smooth paste. Add the cocoa and remaining hot water to the mug, stirring to dissolve.

MAKES 1 SERVING

PER SERVING: 258 calories, 9 g protein, 24 g carbohydrates, 17 g fat, 3 g saturated fat, 8 g monounsaturated fat, 0 mg cholesterol, 4 g fiber, 358 mg sodium

Peanut Butter Creole Soup

Here's a great way to make ordinary canned tomato soup a fast, hearty entrée. If sodium isn't a problem for you, indulge in the regular variety.

  1 can (10½ oz) low-sodium, ready-to-serve tomato
    soup
  2 cups fat-free milk
  ⅔ cup creamy peanut butter
  Tabasco sauce

Combine the soup, milk, and peanut butter in a medium saucepan and warm on medium heat. Stir until the peanut butter melts. Add Tabasco to taste. Serve hot.

MAKES 5 SERVINGS

PER SERVING: 268 calories, 4 g protein, 10 g carbohydrates, 24 g fat, 15 g saturated fat, 7 g monounsaturated fat, 65 mg cholesterol, 0 g fiber, 296 mg sodium

Gingery Peanut-Carrot Soup

Potatoes and peanut butter give this soup its creamy texture. The combo of peanut and carrot flavors, spiced with ginger, is perfect.

  1 Tbsp peanut oil
  1 lb baby carrots
  2 ribs celery, chopped
  1 large white or yellow onion, sliced
  4½ cups water
  2 cups fat-free milk

1 lb baking potatoes, peeled and sliced (about 2 large
    potatoes)
6 Tbsp creamy peanut butter
2 Tbsp minced fresh ginger
1½ tsp salt
1½ tsp white pepper

Place a stockpot over low heat; add the oil, carrots, celery, and onion. Cover and cook, stirring occasionally, for 8 minutes, or until the onions are translucent.

Add the water, milk, potatoes, peanut butter, ginger, salt, and pepper. Cover and bring to a boil. Reduce the heat. Simmer, uncovered, until the veggies are tender, about 25 minutes.

In a blender, puree the soup in batches. Return the soup to the clean stockpot and adjust the seasonings. Heat through over low heat.

MAKES 6 SERVINGS
PER SERVING: 235 calories, 10 g protein, 31 g carbohydrates, 9 g fat, 2 g saturated fat, 4 g monounsaturated fat, 1 mg cholesterol, 4 g fiber, 701 mg sodium

Note: This recipe delivers only 1 Tbsp of peanut butter per serving.

Grilled Peanut Butter and Banana Sandwich

This healthy version of Elvis Presley's favorite peanut butter sandwich is featured at New York's Peanut Butter and Company Restaurant.

8 Tbsp creamy or crunchy peanut butter
8 slices whole grain bread
2 large, ripe bananas, sliced lengthwise into a total of
    16 pieces
2 Tbsp honey

Spread about 1 Tbsp of the peanut butter on each of the bread slices. Place the banana pieces on top of the peanut butter on 4 of the slices and drizzle with the honey. Place the remaining slices of bread on top to make 4 sandwiches.

Place a large, nonstick skillet over medium-high heat. Coat the bread with butter-flavored cooking spray just before browning each side. Sauté (or grill) the sandwiches in batches for approximately 2 minutes per side, or until golden brown. Slice diagonally and serve warm.

MAKES 4 SERVINGS

PER SERVING: 398 calories, 13 g protein, 51 g carbohydrates, 19 g fat, 3 g saturated fat, 8 g monounsaturated fat, 0 mg cholesterol, 9 g fiber, 472 mg sodium

Note: This recipe delivers only 1 Tbsp of peanut butter per serving.

Peanut Butter French Toast

To add a hint of fresh citrus flavor to this breakfast, grate 1 teaspoon of orange peel into the egg batter.

  1 cup Egg Beaters
  ¼ cup fat-free milk
  1 teaspoon vanilla extract
  Dash of salt
  1 Tbsp butter or margarine
  4 slices bread
  ½ cup maple syrup
  ½ cup crunchy peanut butter

In a medium bowl, combine the Egg Beaters, milk, vanilla, and salt. Beat slightly with a fork until blended.

In a medium skillet, melt the butter/margarine. Dip the bread slices into the egg mixture, coating both sides of each. Fry the bread until golden brown on one side; turn and fry the other side.

In a small saucepan, blend the maple syrup and peanut butter. Heat and stir until warm, then pour over the French toast.

MAKES 4 SERVINGS

PER SERVING: 442 calories, 16 g protein, 53 g carbohydrates, 19 g fat, 5 g saturated fat, 9 g monounsaturated fat, 10 mg cholesterol, 3 g fiber, 456 mg sodium

Peanut Butter and Jelly Crackers

Use whole wheat crackers for the most fiber.

   ½ oz whole wheat crackers (e.g., 4 Reduced-Fat
      Triscuits)
   2 Tbsp creamy peanut butter
   1 Tbsp jam or jelly of your choice

Spread half of the crackers with the peanut butter and jelly. Top with the remaining half.

MAKES I SERVING

PER SERVING: 290 calories, 9 g protein, 25 g carbohydrates, 19 g fat, 3 g saturated fat, 8 g monounsaturated fat, 0 mg cholesterol, 4 g fiber, 245 mg sodium

S'Mores

What Peanut Butter Diet would be complete without a version of this childhood campfire favorite? Though most of our recipes combine peanut butter with other good-for-you ingredients, we've included an occasional S'More just for fun.

1 honey graham cracker
2 Tbsp creamy peanut butter
2 Hershey's Kisses
1 Tbsp marshmallow cream (Men's version only)

Spread the graham cracker with the peanut butter and dot with Hershey's Kisses. Men only: top each cracker with the peanut butter and Hershey's Kisses plus 1 Tbsp marshmallow cream.

PER SERVING FOR WOMEN: 300 calories, 10 g protein, 23 g carbohydrates, 21 g fat, 5 g saturated fat, 9 g monounsaturated fat, 2 mg cholesterol, 3 g fiber, 242 mg sodium
PER SERVING FOR MEN: 333 calories, 10 g protein, 31 g carbohydrates, 21 g fat, 5 g saturated fat, 9 g monounsaturated fat, 2 mg cholesterol, 3 g fiber, 242 mg sodium

PB&J on Rye

Look for European whole grain rye in the supermarket deli section. It's dense, moist, and packed with hearty fiber. American "rye" bread uses mostly refined white wheat flour.

1 slice European rye bread
1 Tbsp peanut butter
1 Tbsp jelly or jam of your choice

Spread the bread with the peanut butter and jelly or jam.
MAKES 1 SERVING
PER SERVING: 226 calories, 7 g protein, 32 g carbohydrates, 9 g fat, 1.5 g saturated fat, 4 g monounsaturated fat, 0 mg cholesterol, 3 g fiber, 260 mg sodium

THE PEANUT BUTTER DIET

Homemade Peanut Butter

All you need is a food processor fitted with a steel blade to make the freshest peanut butter possible.

2 cups shelled peanuts

In a food processor fitted with a steel blade, grind the nuts until they produce a spread that's shiny with oil. Occasionally stop the processor to break up the nuts that pack down beneath the blade. Taste the peanut butter to determine that the tex-

> **DID YOU KNOW ...**
>
> Peter Pan peanut butter is the oldest commercial brand.
>
> SOURCE: THE NATIONAL PEANUT BOARD

ture is smooth. Keep refrigerated between uses; it will keep for 2 weeks or longer.

MAKES I CUP (I6 TBSP)

PER 2 TBSP: 212 calories, 10 g protein, 6 g carbohydrate, 18 g fat, 3 g saturated fat, 8 g monounsaturated fat, 0 mg cholesterol, 2 g fiber, 2 mg sodium

Peanut Butter–Maple Syrup Waffles

Frozen waffles make instant platforms for peanut butter breakfast treats.

2 whole grain frozen waffles
2 Tbsp peanut butter
3 tsp maple syrup
1 small banana, sliced

Toast the waffles and spread each with 1 Tbsp of the peanut butter. Top each with 1 tsp of the maple syrup and half of the banana slices.

MAKES I SERVING
PER SERVING: 520 calories, 16 g protein, 23 g carbohydrates, 26 g fat, 6.6 g saturated fat, 11 g monounsaturated fat, 75 mg cholesterol, 8 g fiber, 436 mg sodium.

Peanut Butter Banana

This classic, satisfying snack fulfills more than 20 percent of your daily potassium needs. This mineral helps keep your blood vessels relaxed and protects you from stroke.

1 banana
2 Tbsp peanut butter

Slice the banana lengthwise. Spread the inside of 1 slice with the peanut butter, then top with the other slice.
MAKES I SERVING
PER SERVING: 297 calories, 9 g protein, 35 g carbohydrates, 17 g fat, 3.3 g saturated fat, 8 g monounsaturated fat, 0 mg cholesterol, 5 g fiber, 157 mg sodium

Peanut Butter Bagel

Simply by replacing the cream cheese on your bagel with peanut butter, you lose 3 grams of artery-clogging saturated fat and gain 5 grams of artery-cleaning monounsaturated fat—plus vitamins and minerals galore. Try an onion bagel for big flavor.

2 Tbsp peanut butter
½ small (2 oz) bagel

Spread the peanut butter on the bagel half.
MAKES I SERVING

PER SERVING: 303 calories, 13 g protein, 30 g carbohydrate, 17 g fat, 3 g saturated fat, 8 g monounsaturated fat, 0 mg cholesterol, 4 g fiber, 375 mg sodium

---

Beware of monster bagels. Today, the "average" bagel is actually double what it would have been 20 years ago. If you have a 4-oz bagel (equal to 4 slices of bread!), use only ¼ of it for this snack.

CHAPTER FOURTEEN

Customize the 4-Week Plan

As with hats, no diet is truly "one size fits all." So I've come up with what I think are the three most likely reasons that the Peanut Butter Diet may not fit you to a tee. And I've found ways that you can tweak it to make it fit, no matter what.

1. YOU NEED A BREAK FROM PEANUT BUTTER

Suppose you try the Peanut Butter Diet, and, like the people in the study described in chapter 2, you find losing weight and keeping it off to be easier on a calorie-controlled eating plan that's rich in good-for-you monounsaturated fat. You get more pleasure and satisfaction from your food than you did when you tried a low-fat, high-carbohydrate diet.

But then you realize that you're getting tired of eating peanut butter twice a day, every day. I expect that even the most diehard peanut butter fanatic will eventually reach that point, after being able to indulge those peanut butter cravings without guilt for a while.

If you find yourself in this situation, you're probably ready to change your diet so that you get your monounsaturated fat from foods other than peanut butter. You can create your own satisfying, peanut-butter-free menus us-

MONOUNSATURATED FAT DIET FORMULA

Whether you need a break from peanut butter or you want to create new peanut butter menus, this chart can help you do it. Just make sure you're getting the right number of servings from each food group, based on 1,500 calories if you're a woman or 2,200 calories if you're a man.

FOOD GROUP	PORTION	MENU PLAN FOR WOMEN (1,500 CALORIES)	MENU PLAN FOR MEN (2,200 CALORIES)
Monounsaturated fats	½ tsp peanut butter; 1½ tsp tree nut butters such as almond or cashew butter; 1 tsp olive, canola, or peanut oil; ⅛ tsp avocado; 1 Tbsp peanuts; 1 Tbsp tree nuts, such as macadamias or pecans	13 servings	17 servings
Fruits	1 small piece, ½ cup cut fruit, ¾ cup fruit juice (especially calcium-enriched citrus juice), ¼ cup dried fruit	3 servings	3 servings
Vegetables	1 cup salad greens, ½ cup other vegetables, ¾ cup vegetable juice (especially calcium-enriched V8)	6 servings	6 servings
Whole grains and potatoes	1 slice bread, ½ cup rice or pasta, ½ cup potatoes, 1 serving whole grain breakfast cereal	3 servings	7 servings
Calcium-rich foods	1 cup fat-free or 1% milk, 1 cup fat-free yogurt, 1 oz reduced-fat cheese, fat-free calcium-enriched soy milk	2 servings*	2 servings*
Lean proteins	1 oz lean meat, poultry, or fish; ½ cup cooked legumes	4 servings	8 servings

*To meet their bodies' calcium needs, people under age 50 should either take a 300-milligram calcium supplement or ¾ cup of calcium-enriched V8 or citrus juice daily (This counts as one veggie or fruit serving). People 50 and older also have two choices: a 500-milligram supplement or a 300-milligram supplement *plus* ¾ cup of calcium-enriched juice daily.

ing the Monounsaturated Fat Diet Formula on page 206. It organizes foods into six groups and indicates the number of servings from each group that will yield a menu providing 1,500 calories for women and 2,200 calories for men. A rich 35 percent of those calories come from mostly monounsaturated fat. Following the formula, women get 13 servings of foods from the monounsaturated fat group; men get 17 servings. If you want to create menus without peanut butter, just don't choose it for any of your servings. You can replace it with avocados, pecans, cashews, almond butter, olive oil, and many other mouthwatering foods rich in monounsaturated fat.

On the other hand, if your peanut butter tooth isn't satisfied by the menu plans and recipes I've provided, you can use the formula to design your own peanut butter menu. If you're a woman, you'll want eight of your monounsaturated fat servings to come from peanut butter, for 4 tablespoons total. Men should aim for 12 servings of peanut butter, or 6 tablespoons total. That's exactly how we created the Peanut Butter Diet menu plans in chapters 11 and 12.

2. YOU'RE GETTING TOO MANY CALORIES

The menu plans for women are designed to provide 1,500 calories a day. Based on that intake, most women should be able to lose weight at the moderate but healthy pace of about ½ pound a week. (Remember, though, that if you want to slim down, you must also accumulate 45 minutes of activity every day. You'll read more about exercise in chapter 15.)

In general, *Prevention* magazine does not recommend that women cut calories any lower. On so little food, you feel deprived, which could help set you up to start over-

PEANUT BUTTER DIET FORMULA
FOR PETITE WOMEN

If the 1,500 calories in the menu plans for women is too much for you, you can create your own 1,200-calorie menu by following this chart. Just choose the specified number of servings from each food group.

FOOD GROUP	PORTION	MENU PLAN (1,200 CALORIES)
Monoun-saturated fats	½ tsp peanut butter; 1½ tsp tree nut butters such as almond or cashew butter; 1 tsp olive, canola, or peanut oil; 1/8 avocado; 1 Tbsp peanuts; 1 Tbsp tree nuts, such as macadamias or pecans	8 servings of peanut butter daily (4 table spoons total) plus 2 servings of other high-mono foods
Fruits	1 small piece, ½ cup cut fruit, ¾ cup fruit juice (especially calcium-enriched citrus juice), ¼ cup dried fruit	3 servings
Vegetables	1 cup salad greens, ½ cup other vegetables, ¾ cup vegetable juice (especially calcium-enriched V8)	5 servings
Whole grains and potatoes	1 slice bread, ½ cup rice or pasta, ½ cup potatoes, 1 serving whole grain breakfast cereal	3 servings
Calcium-rich foods	1 cup fat-free or 1% milk, 1 cup fat-free yogurt, 1 oz reduced-fat cheese, or fat-free calcium-enriched soy milk	1 serving*
Lean protein	1 oz lean meat, poultry, or fish; ½ cup cooked legumes	2 servings

*To meet their bodies' calcium needs, women under age 50 should take a 300-milligram calcium supplement and drink ¾ cup calcium-enriched citrus juice or V8 as one fruit or veggie serving. Women 50 and older should take a 500-milligram calcium supplement and drink ¾ cup calcium-enriched citrus juice or V8 as one fruit or veggie serving.

SKIP THE PEANUT BUTTER, NOT THE BENEFITS

For women, a mono-rich menu plan without peanut butter might look something like this.

Breakfast: I cup raisin bran; I Tbsp roasted almonds; I cup strawberries; I cup fat-free milk

Lunch: Open-face sandwich made with ¼ sliced avocado, ½ tomato, ½ cup shredded carrots, and I cup romaine lettuce drizzled with I tsp olive oil, all on I slice whole wheat bread

Snack: 2 Tbsp cashew butter spread on slices of I apple

Dinner: 4 oz. broiled salmon; ½ cup whole wheat pasta with I Tbsp olive oil, I Tbsp balsamic vinegar, I cup broccoli florets, and ½ cup califlower

Evening treat: 2 Tbsp roasted pecans mixed in 8 oz fat-free strawberry yogurt

The men's version would supply more calories—2,200, compared with 1,500 for women.

Breakfast: I cup raisin bran; I Tbsp roasted almonds; I cup strawberries; I cup fat-free milk

Lunch: Sandwich made with 4 oz sliced turkey, ¼ sliced avocado, ½ tomato, ½ cup shredded carrots drizzled with I tsp olive oil, all on 2 slices whole wheat bread

Snack: 2 Tbsp cashew butter spread on slices of I apple

Dinner: 4 oz. broiled salmon; ½ cup whole wheat pasta with 2 Tbsp olive oil, 2 Tbsp balsamic vinegar, I cup broccoli florets, and ½ cup califlower

Evening treat: 2 Tbsp roasted pecans mixed in 8 oz fat-free strawberry yogurt

eating again. What's more, when the pounds come off too fast, you end up shedding not just fat but calorie-burning muscle.

The sole exceptions to the calorie-cutting rule are women who are very petite—5 feet 2 inches or smaller. If you're in this category, you probably won't be able to slim down on 1,500 calories a day. You may want to try

TRIM CALORIES—AND POUNDS!

Here's an example of a peanut butter menu plan that provides just 1,200 calories. *Prevention* magazine recommends this type of plan *only* for petite women who are not able to lose weight on 1,500 calories a day.

Breakfast: ½ toasted English muffin spread with 2 Tbsp peanut butter; ½ cup berries; 1 cup fat-free milk

Lunch: Salad made with 2 oz chicken breast, ½ tomato, ½ cup shredded carrots, and 1 cup romaine lettuce, drizzled with 2 tsp olive oil and 1 tsp balsamic vinegar; ¾ cup calcium-enriched orange juice

Snack: Small banana, spread with 1 Tbsp peanut butter

Dinner: 1 cup whole wheat pasta with ½ cup pasta sauce; 1 cup broccoli florets; ½ cup sliced cucumbers in vinegar

Evening treat: 1 Tbsp melted peanut butter on ½ cup fat-free frozen yogurt

building your own peanut-buttery menu plans so they provide just 1,200 calories a day—but with 35 percent of those calories still coming from healthy monounsaturated fat. Just follow the Peanut Butter Diet Formula for Petite Women on the page 208. It's a modification of the Monounsaturated Fat Diet Formula.

If you go with the 1,200-calorie menus, you should also take a daily multivitamin/mineral supplement. It can help make up for any potential nutritional shortfalls.

3. YOU WANT TO EAT OUT

One of the reasons the Peanut Butter Diet works is that all the meals and snacks without peanut butter are designed to be low in calories. That's why you can eat your 4 or 6 tablespoons of calorie-dense peanut butter and still lose weight.

But what happens when you need to grab lunch at McDonalds or Denny's? Or you're joining friends for dinner at a new Italian trattoria? It's really pretty simple: Whenever you eat out, you make a commitment to fol-

> **DID YOU KNOW . . .**
>
> About 1 in every 10 peanuts grown for food in the United States ends up in a jar of Jif brand peanut butter.
>
> SOURCE: THE NATIONAL PEANUT BOARD

low these Rules of Restaurant Survival. They'll let you enjoy your meal while controlling your calorie intake—with enough calories left over for your two scrumptious peanut butter treats!

1. Always order the smallest size, even when the restaurant has a special deal on the jumbo burger or monster fries. Otherwise, you'll save money but lose your figure.
2. Eat only half, or less, of your entrée or deli sandwich. Portions in American restaurants have become so humongous that you can easily blow an entire day's calorie budget on one meal if you clean your plate. Don't.
3. Have no more than two slices of pizza. Ask for light cheese, extra tomato sauce, and lots of onions and mushrooms.
4. Instead of high-calorie soft drinks, have zero-calorie club soda, seltzer, mineral water, or plain iced tea. Or quench your thirst for free with ice water.
5. Skip appetizers, except shrimp or crab cocktail. Pass up those little cups of cream soup that ooze calories. Instead, fill up on a tossed salad. Always order dressing on the side, then use the dip-spear method: Dip your fork in the dressing, then spear a hunk of lettuce or piece of tomato.

6. Ask the waiter to take away the bread basket.
7. Avoid anything that's fried. If a dish comes with cream, cheese, or butter sauce, ask for the sauce on the side and use the dip-spear method. If a dish is described as "topped with cheese," tell the waiter you want only a little cheese, about the size of an Oreo cookie.
8. Unless you can order fresh berries or other fruit, skip dessert. (Sorry, no peanut butter pie. The healthy peanut butter comes with a ton of extra calories from pastry shortening, cream, and sugar.) Sip coffee or tea while your fellow diners indulge. Remind yourself how fabulous and filling your peanut butter treat will taste when you get home.

Don't worry about getting your calories to balance out exactly. You won't be able to, especially when you decide to eat out on the spur of the moment. The Rules of Restaurant Survival will help rein in your calorie intake. You may have noticed that some of the menu plans in chapters 11 and 12 already include low-calorie restaurant choices.

As long as you keep your meal low-cal, you can still enjoy two luscious peanut butter dishes. To reward yourself for being good, make sure you select at least one of your favorite treats—maybe a Peanut Butter Sundae (page 192)?—and enjoy it without guilt. In fact, while you're at the restaurant, picture that peanut butter treat waiting for you and imagine how luscious it will taste. That just may keep you from overindulging!

CHAPTER FIFTEEN

Don't Forget Your Vitamin X

If you want to slim down—with the Peanut Butter Diet or any other diet—you've got to get moving. In other words, you have to get more vitamin X, as in "x-ercise." To help you achieve the weight-loss results you want, I'm going to show you how you need to move, how *much* you need to move, and how to fit fitness into the busiest lifestyle, especially if you're the type who's "allergic" to exercise.

The reality is, most of us struggle daily to find balance between increasing opportunities to eat high-calorie foods and decreasing opportunities to burn off those extra calories. We sit constantly—in cars, behind desks, at doctors' offices. We no longer rake leaves; we blow them. We don't push lawn mowers; we ride them. We don't get up to change the channel on the TV; we click a button. We don't even turn on the faucets in public restrooms; we hold out our hands, and the water starts flowing as if by magic.

> **DID YOU KNOW ...**
>
> Skippy peanut butter has outsold every other brand in the world.
>
> SOURCE: THE NATIONAL PEANUT BOARD

In short, we're using up fewer calories on a daily basis. What happens to all the extras we're consuming? They turn to fat. No wonder more than half of all Americans are now overweight—and the number keeps rising every year.

Health authorities believe that by itself, controlling calories is not enough to stem the epidemic of obesity.

That's why the U.S. government's updated dietary guidelines, issued in 2000, advise adults interested in losing weight or maintaining weight loss to accumulate 45 minutes of physical activity every day.

LOOK WHAT ELSE EXERCISE CAN DO

For many people, the promise of lasting weight loss just might be enough to kick-start a fitness routine. But exercise can do so much more for the body and mind. Here are some examples.

It protects against heart attack. Like all muscles, the heart responds to physical activity by becoming stronger and more efficient.

It takes down cholesterol. In particular, exercise reduces LDL cholesterol, the bad kind that forms artery-clogging plaque and contributes to high blood pressure, heart attacks, and strokes. It also increases HDL, the good cholesterol.

It fights diabetes. By enabling muscles to take up blood sugar and use it as energy, working out helps keep blood sugar and insulin levels on an even keel. This is how exercise can help prevent diabetes—or control it, if you already have it.

It builds strong bones. Lifetime walkers are less likely to develop osteoporosis. What's more, strength training can help increase bone density.

It prevents colon cancer. Exercise speeds digested food through the colon, denying potential carcinogens the opportunity to affect the colon lining.

It safeguards against breast cancer. By reducing body fat, physical activity reduces the production of estrogen, which promotes some types of breast cancer.

It improves your mood. Most people feel a sense of calm and well-being after working out, probably due in part to the release of beta-endorphins, the body's natural mood enhancers. This benefit kicks in as soon as 12 minutes after an exercise session.

SUCCESSFUL LOSERS PROVE IT WORKS

While most experts agree that slimming down through exercise alone is difficult, they also feel that physical activity—along with calorie control—is essential to any weight-loss program. In fact, in a four-year study involving 20,000 men, researchers at Brigham and Women's Hospital in Boston found that exercise was the single strongest predictor of weight loss or gain.

Even more important, increasing your daily dose of vitamin X may be the ticket to keeping off pounds for good, which is the hardest part of any slim-down plan. Through his work with the National Weight Control Registry, a database of more 3,000 Americans who have lost at least 30 pounds and maintained the loss for at least a year, codirector James Hill, Ph.D., has observed that long-term weight maintenance is rare without regular exercise. Most successful maintainers, he says, work out for the equivalent of walking an hour a day. And compared with the general population, these people are much more likely to lift weights.

HOW TO LEAP THE TIME BARRIER

I can guess what you're thinking right now, because I often think the same thing: "Forty-five minutes of physical activity a day? Impossible!" Yet if we truly want to take pounds off and keep them off, we must change our mindset to "How can I make those 45 minutes happen?"

This is where a little myth-busting comes in handy. It makes those 45 minutes seem a lot more doable—so much so that I remind myself of it almost every day. It really helps.

What is the myth? That exercise counts only when it's done all at once.

In a national survey, 47 percent of Americans cited lack of time as their biggest obstacle to regular physical activity. No wonder! Carving a 45-minute chunk out of most people's crazy schedules is ridiculously unrealistic. Yet most of us believe it's the only way that a workout will make a difference.

Now for the wonderful news: Many studies have shown that accumulating 45 minutes of activity in several short spurts over the course of a day may be just as effective for weight loss as exercising for one long 45-minute session. Perhaps the short spurts work because they're much easier to fit into your day—and not nearly so daunting.

In one 20-week study, 56 women—all considered obese—were assigned to one of two groups. The "long-bout" group was instructed to engage in a single extended workout daily, starting with 20-minute sessions and advancing to 40-minute sessions. The "short-bout" group was told to exercise in

> **QUICK TIP**
>
> Some activity—even just 5 minutes a day—is much better than no activity at all.

multiple 10-minute spurts throughout the day, aiming for a total of 20 minutes of activity to start and working up to a total of 40 minutes. In addition, all of the women followed eating plans that provided between 1,200 and 1,500 calories per day.

The results? The short-bout group reported exercising on 87 days, versus 69 days for the long-bout group. The short-bout group accumulated 224 minutes of exercise a week, compared with the long-bout group, which got only 188 minutes. The short-bout group lost an average of 9 pounds; the long-bout group lost an average of 6 pounds. The researchers concluded that exercising in spurts had increased adherence. And isn't adherence—sticking with it—the key to an effective fitness regimen and successful weight loss? You bet.

Other studies have shown that people burn more calories in one continuous workout session than in several short bouts. But in my mind, if doing a little at a time enables you to exercise longer and more consistently, then short bouts seem like your best choice.

What's more, much research concludes that exercising in spurts improves cardiovascular fitness and decreases blood pressure as much as working out in longer sessions. In one study, walking for 5 minutes at a time, with a goal of accumulating 30 minutes over the course of the day, was as effective as walking for 30 minutes all at once.

THE DEFINITION OF EXERCISE? NOT SITTING

So what constitutes exercise? Most of us are still stuck in the rut of thinking that we need to climb on a treadmill or stair climber, enroll in an aerobics class, sign up for an official "walk" or "run." In fact, a survey found that 66 percent of Americans agreed with this statement: "If you don't raise a sweat when exercising, you're probably not exercising hard enough for it to do much good."

But as the chart on page 218 shows, you can burn a surprising number of calories in just 10 minutes of some very ordinary, day-to-day activities—things like vacuuming, scrubbing the tub, and mowing the lawn. I hope the chart gets you thinking about the many different ways you can "exercise" just by engaging in short bouts of a variety of activities on a daily basis. And don't focus solely on calorie burn. Some experts suspect that it's not how much time you spend engaging in vigorous, sweat-inducing workouts that matters. Rather, it's how much

---

A LITTLE EXERCISE MEANS A LOT

You don't need a formal fitness regimen to shape up and slim down. As the following chart shows, even routine activities help use up calories over the course of a day. The right-hand column shows the number of calories that a 150-pound woman would burn in 10 minutes of each activity.

ACTIVITY	CALORIES BURNED
Stair-stepping	102
Swimming laps (freestyle, slow pace)	79
Aerobic dancing (moderate effort)	74
Mowing the lawn (push power mower)	62
Stationary bicycling (light effort)	62
Aerobic dancing (low-impact)	57
Carrying a load up stairs (1 to 15 lb)	57
Basketball (shooting baskets)	51
Line dancing	51
Raking leaves	49
Bicycling (less than 10 mph)	45
Caring for an elderly disabled person (active periods only)	45
Sweeping the sidewalk	45
Scrubbing the bathtub	43
Golf (using a power cart)	40
Vacuuming	40
Walking (for pleasure; work break)	40
Dressing, feeding, or lifting a child (standing)	34
Painting walls	34
Walking the dog	34
Playing with children (standing)	32
Light cleaning (dusting, straightening up)	28
Mowing the lawn (riding mower)	28
Food shopping (standing or walking)	26
Making the bed	23

time you spend not being totally inactive—glued to the computer or the TV, for example.

Imagine a day where your "workout" consists of the following activities.

- Spending 10 minutes on the treadmill before you shower and dress
- Walking 5 minutes from the parking lot to your workplace
- Going outside for a 10-minute walk before you eat lunch (or, if the weather is nasty, staying inside and walking around your workplace, including up and down the stairs)
- Walking 5 minutes back to your car to head for home
- Scrubbing the tub for 5 minutes while dinner is cooking
- Dancing to your favorite salsa CD for 10 minutes after dinner

That adds up to the recommended 45 minutes of activity a day. Does it seem doable? Absolutely! It's much better than being completely inactive.

If you get to a point where you feel motivated to try longer sessions of an activity you especially enjoy, go for it! You may burn more calories, and if you really love what you're doing, you have a great chance of sticking with it. Until you reach that point, however, my vote is for accumulating exercise in short bouts. Personally, I find it's a much better fit for my current lifestyle and motivation level.

THE SECRET TO BURNING CALORIES WHILE YOU SLEEP

Most of the activities listed on page 218 are the aerobic kind, meaning that they get your heart pumping faster. More and more research shows that another type of activity, strength training, is just as crucial to your weight-loss efforts. It melts away pounds while toning and sculpting your body, so you look fantastic.

Do you know what finally got me started lifting weights? I learned that strength training enables my body to burn more calories—not just while I'm working out but 24 hours a day.

The reason is pure physiology. To sustain a pound of fat for a day, your body spends a measly 2 calories, says Wayne Westcott, Ph.D., strength-training consultant for the American Senior Fitness Association in New Smyrna Beach, Florida. That's next to nothing! By contrast, sustaining a pound of muscle for a day requires 30 calories.

So let's say you replace just 2 pounds of fat with 2 pounds of muscle. That means that every day, even while you sleep, your body would burn as many as 60 extra calories just to keep you alive. Within a year, you'd lose more than 6 pounds. That's what I call sweet dreams!

YOU'RE NEVER TOO OLD TO BUILD MUSCLE

By now you may be thinking: "Lift weights? At my age?" You bet! The fact is, the older you get, the more important building muscle becomes. "One of the big reasons most people put on weight as they age is that their activity level declines and their muscle mass decreases," explains my colleague Michele Stanten, *Prevention* magazine's fitness editor. In fact, most folks lose ¼ to ½ pound of muscle each year, replacing it with fat. For women in menopause, the rate of muscle loss jumps to about 1 pound a year.

So even if you're eating about the same as you did in your twenties, you're burning fewer calories because your muscles are getting smaller. No wonder the pounds creep on. "If you want to prevent that, the smartest strategy is to start lifting weights," Stanten advises.

Granted, aerobic activities burn more calories while you're doing them. And they have important benefits for your heart and lungs. But as Stanten points out, aerobic exercise usually doesn't build muscle, and the calorie burning lasts only a short time after your workout ends.

On the other hand, strength training increases muscle mass, which means you're burning more calories every second of the day—even while you sleep. It's the only metabolism booster that really works.

AFRAID YOU'LL LOOK LIKE MR. UNIVERSE?

Another common deterrent to lifting weights, especially among women, is a fear of bulking up like Arnold Schwarzenegger. If this is one of your concerns, you can cross it off your list right now.

Unlike the male body, the female body is not genetically programmed to develop heavily defined muscles, Stanten explains. We've all seen female weight lifters with muscular physiques. But fitness experts suggest that these women are likely to be taking anabolic steroids, a very dangerous practice.

Another factor that determines how much you bulk up is how much you train. According to Stanten, competitive body builders spend hours at the gym every day. For the sleek, firm look most women long for, the best results come from two or three 20-minute workouts a week. And for most women, one set of 8 to 12 repetitions of each exercise will be enough. This increases muscle mass, but in a way that provides an overall toned look.

If you've never tried strength training, you'll be amazed at how quickly your body responds to it. You should notice a difference in less than a month.

PUT AWAY THE SCALE FOR GOOD

The best measure of your weight-loss success is not your scale but your clothes, particularly if you're doing any sort of strength training. If you find that you can zip up your slacks or buckle your belt more easily than before, you've got proof positive that you're moving in the right direction, even if your scale has hardly budged.

The reason? Muscle weighs more than fat. In fact, a handful of muscle tissue is 22 percent heavier than an equal amount of fat. So as you build muscle mass through strength training, your scale won't show the results. (It might even inch upward!) But because muscle takes up less space than fat—and looks a heck of a lot better, too—your clothes will instantly tell you what you've accomplished.

And remember: A pound of muscle burns about 15 times more calories a day than a pound of fat. And that burn occurs even while you sleep!

GET STARTED WITH THE BASIC SIX

You don't need to join a gym to reap the benefits of weight lifting (although it's a good place to start if you'd like some personal training in proper form and technique). To make your workout as efficient as possible, Stanten—who's certified by the American Council on Exercise—has selected six fundamental exercises that you can do in your own home. They'll work your muscles just enough to improve strength and tone. You can always add more exercises, if you wish. You'll have a fabulous foundation to build on.

While the Basic Six work all of your body's major muscle groups, you'll notice that most of the exercises concentrate on the upper body—your shoulders, arms, chest, and back. That's for a very practical reason. "Most daily activities involve your leg muscles," Stanten explains. "So does most aerobic exercise, like stepping or dancing. Most women and even lots of guys don't work their upper-body muscles. If you do these six exercises, you'll be using muscles you might not have challenged in years."

The Gear
The Basic Six do require some basic equipment. Here's what you need.

Dumbbells. Also called free weights, these are available in 1-pound increments from 1 to 20 pounds. Pairs of 3-, 5-, 8-, and 10-pound dumbbells should be sufficient. You'll pay between $25 and $55 for all four pairs at a sporting goods store.

Comfortable clothes. No sexy leotards necessary! You want to choose an outfit that's breathable but not so baggy that it interferes with your movements. You might even try a pair of pajamas. Be sure to wear your athletic shoes, too. They make you more stable, and they'll protect your feet better than most shoes should you drop a dumbbell.

The Workout
Once you have your equipment, you're all set to start lifting. Just follow these guidelines to keep your strength-

training sessions safe—and to give your muscles an optimum workout.

Warm up first. Before you pick up those dumbbells, you need to prime your muscles for exertion. Walking or jogging in place for at least 5 minutes should do the trick.

Choose the right weight. You should be able to lift your dumbbells 8 to 12 times while maintaining good form. In other words, you can perform the required movements smoothly, without shaking too much as you finish your last repetitions (or reps, in gym-speak). If you can't do at least 8 reps with good form, switch to a lighter weight.

On the other hand, if you can easily do more than 12 repetitions, your dumbbells are too light, in which case you can move up to the next heavier weight. You should feel some muscle fatigue after doing 10 to 12 repetitions. Remember, muscles change only when you challenge them.

Do the reps. Do 8 to 12 repetitions, or one set, of each exercise per session.

Take your time. Each repetition should last about 6 seconds. Slowly count "1–2–3" as you lift the weight and "1–2–3" as you lower it.

Skip a day. Do the Basic Six two or three times a week, but not on consecutive days. Your muscles need a day's rest in between.

The Exercises
Ready to try the Basic Six? Just follow the instructions below.

THE IMPORTANCE OF BEING A BREATHER

I've always found the descriptions for breathing properly while lifting weights very confusing. The experts say to inhale as you lower the weights with gravity and exhale as you lift against it. My translation: Breathe in on the part of the exercise that's easiest, and breathe out on the part that requires the most work.

What if you forget to breathe that way? Is the exercise worthless? Absolutely not! The most important thing is to remember to breathe, period. For some reason, people tend to hold their breath when they're lifting weights. That can cause blood pressure to spike. However, counting aloud as you lift ("2–3" on the way up, "1–2–3" on the way down) ensures that you're not holding your breath and keeps your blood pressure on an even keel.

1. **Chest press:** This exercise works the muscles in your chest. Lying face-up on the floor, hold the dumbbells end-to-end right above your chest with your palms facing forward. Lower your arms until your elbows, which should be pointing out to the sides, touch the floor. Return to the starting position, then repeat 8 to 12 times.

2. **Squat:** This exercise works the muscles in your buttocks and legs. Stand with your back against a wall with a dumbbell in each hand. Slide down the wall as if you were sitting in a chair, going only to the point where your thighs are parallel to the floor and no farther. Be sure your knees don't move forward over your toes. Keep

QUICK TIP

Always remember to protect your back. When you pick up your weights from the floor, squat and lift with your legs, rather than bending forward and lifting with your back.

your head up and facing forward, your shoulders back, and your back straight. Return to the starting position and repeat 8 to 12 times.

3. Bent-over row: This exercise works the muscles in your upper back. Stand next to a sturdy chair. Bending at the hips, place your left hand on the chair seat. Holding a dumbbell in your right hand, let your arm hang straight down with your palm facing the chair. Keep your back flat and parallel to the floor. Pull the dumbbell up toward your chest. Hold, then lower. Repeat 8 to 12 times with your right arm, then switch to your left.

4. Overhead press: This exercise works the muscles in your shoulders as well as your triceps, the "floppy" muscles under the upper arms that many women want to tone. Holding a dumbbell in each hand, stand with your feet shoulder-width apart. Position the dumbbells at shoulder height, with your palms facing in. Lift the dumbbells straight up overhead, then lower them to shoulder height. Repeat 8 to 12 times, making sure not to arch your back.

5. Biceps curl: This exercise works your biceps, the muscles on the front of the upper arms. With a dumbbell in each hand, stand with your feet shoulder-width apart. Hold the weights at your sides, with your palms facing your legs. Keeping your elbows close to your waist, lift the dumbbells toward your chest. As you do, turn your hands so that when the weights get to chest height, your palms are facing your chest. Return the dumbbells to your sides. Repeat 8 to 12 times.

6. Chest lift: This exercise works the muscles of your lower back. Lie face-down on the floor with your hands underneath your chin. Lift your head and chest about 5 inches off the floor, then slowly lower. Repeat 8 to 12 times.